MASSAGING your Baby

THE JOY OF TOUCH TIME

DR. ELAINE FOGEL SCHNEIDER

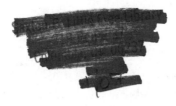

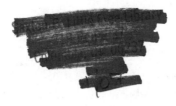

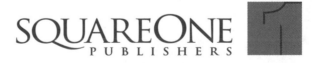

SQUAREONE
PUBLISHERS

Before beginning a massage, the author and publisher recommend that you check the contraindications (cautions) on page 43. Always seek the advice of your healthcare provider before massaging your baby. Neither the author nor the publisher can be held responsible for any damage or injury resulting from the use of baby massage or any of the advice or recommendations in this book.

The rhymes and songs appearing on pages 107 to 124 are copyrighted by Dr. Elaine Fogel Schneider.

TouchTime is a registered trademark belonging to Dr. Elaine Fogel Schneider.

Cover Designer: Jacqueline Michelus and Jeannie Tudor
Typesetter: Gary A. Rosenberg
Cover Photo: Edo Tsoar
Interior Photos: Edo Tsoar and Karen B. Christy (see Photo Credits on page 206)
Editor: Elaine Weiser

Square One Publishers
115 Herricks Road
Garden City Park, NY 11040
(516) 535-2010 • (877) 900-BOOK
www.squareonepublishers.com

Library of Congress Cataloging-in-Publication Data
Schneider, Elaine Fogel.
    Massaging your baby : the joy of touch time / Elaine Fogel Schneider.
        p. cm.
    Includes bibliographical references and index.
    ISBN 0-7570-0263-3 (pbk.)
1. Massage for infants. I. Title.

RJ53.M35S34 2005
649'.4—dc22

2005031329

Printed in the United States of America

10   9   8   7   6   5   4   3   2   1

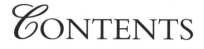

CONTENTS

*This book is dedicated
to the loving touches of
my husband, Jack, and daughter, Karli,
my parents,
and families everywhere*

$\mathcal{P}$REFACE

Welcome to the world of parenting and relationships. You may know the saying, "No man is an island unto himself" and I might add, "Neither is a baby!" When I first started studying in the field of child development, at Hunter College City University of New York in 1963, it was just that . . . all about the CHILD. Later, I studied and taught at Queens College City University of New York, in 1969, and after being a speech and language pathologist, teacher of the deaf and hard of hearing, and a professional dancer and dance teacher, I ventured into the dance/movement field at New York University, in 1975. Here I was able to piece together the non-verbal and verbal worlds of a child, learning more about movement, the body, and the mind. Working in the fields of communication, infant mental health, early intervention, and infant massage, I feel that I have come "home" to appreciate the phenomenal physiological, emotional, and cognitive growth of infants within the one place they come "home" to, and that is their family.

I am so excited by the recent brilliant and dedicated work of researchers from all different walks of life, shedding light on infancy, relationships, the brain, and emotions. Physicians, neurologists, psychiatrists, psychologists, educators, infant mental health professionals, and biologists are discovering new evidence of how babies grow and learn, notwithstanding how touch has far-reaching effects on well-being. No longer is infancy seen as a time for sleeping and resting after the long "trip" down the birth canal. It is seen as a time of memory making, establishing secure attachments, growing brains in structure and function, pruning excess dendrites, and forming relationships, which will affect all future relationships.

When a baby is not touched, he can wither and die, or his brain will be smaller than the brain of another child who is nurtured; massage a depressed mom who has a depressed baby and both will improve their emotional states. TouchTime promotes wellness in your child and yourself, for it brings two willing beings together in a moment of time, when nothing else matters in the world but reading your baby's cues and following your baby's lead through the natural communicator, the first language of touch.

No book can be published without the great assistance of those who believe in the message of your word. I want to take this opportunity to thank my dear, sweet husband of twenty-eight years, Jack, and our wonderful daughter Karli who support me with their nurturing love, touches, and kindness. Also, Rudy Shur of Square One Publishers for giving me this opportunity to publish this work, Lisa Messinger, my dear friend and "guide," and Elaine Weiser, editor, who gave so much to this labor of love. (Having the same first name was also fun.) My mother, brother, stepdaughter Cyndy Fischer, and other family members and friends are thanked for their ongoing encouragement. Susan Ram brought me the additional parent perspective and was a second pair of eyes. Diane Mayer nurtured my body and mind by being the best massage therapist ever, Thelma Lager provided extraordinary wisdom, and Karen B. Christy visually captured the loving massages of many families whom you will meet in this book.

I would like to acknowledge Carlos Flores, who provided me the opportunity of demonstrating infant massage on a Public Service Announcement for the State of California's Department of Developmental Disabilities Early Start program, which validated infant massage as a therapeutic intervention for early intervention programs everywhere. Dr. Joel Stark at Queens College, in 1967, taught me that getting down to a child's level did not mean to cognitively get down to their level, but to physically get down on the floor, when all the therapists I knew sat in chairs. I am eternally grateful to Mother Teresa, for inspiring kindness and compassion with her healing touch, and I give thanks to all my instructors in the Dance Therapy Department at New York University who were teaching about the mind/body connection and touch before it was fashionable.

I value all the families who shared their stories, and all of the families I have worked with over these thirty-five years. I value the compassionate medical professionals Drs. Feldman and Salomonson who revealed the depth of their commitment to touch, healing, and the well-being of their patients.

I would like to acknowledge Margie Wagner for her graciousness and believing in TouchTime, Kalena Babeshoff for being a compassionate teacher and friend in my world of infant massage, and the many other friends and professionals from across so many disciplines who have contributed to my learning. Ashley Montagu, Connie Lillas, Alan Schore, Daniel J. Siegel, Jeree Pawl, T. Berry Brazelton, Stanley Greenspan, Ed Tronick, Bruce Perry, Emily Fenichel, Kathryn Barnard, Bob Jacobs, Heidi Als, Tiffany Field and the Touch Research Institute, Saul Schanberg, Harry Harlow, Rene Spitz, John Bowlby, Marshall Klaus, John Kennell, and other researchers, recent or long gone, whose works have inspired us to look at infants and children after seeing the value of touch with our mammalian friends. I also am thankful for Deepak Chopra and Candace Pert for being beautiful pioneers in the field of body/mind connections, and Vimala McClure, for bringing infant massage to the West. All of the State of California's Interagency Coordinating Council members and community representatives, in addition to the staffs of the Department of Developmental Services for the State of California, California Department of Education, WestEd-CPEI, Zero to Three, Infant Development Association, Family Focus Resource Centers, Kaiser Permanente Health Care Systems, and North Los Angeles County Regional Center staffs, including George Stevens, Susana Gil, Jennifer Kaiser, Raymond "Mac" Peterson, Rick Ingraham, Cheri Schoenborn, Marie Kanne Paulsen, Arlene Downing, Beverly Morgan-Sandoz, Jim Bellotti, Zelna Banks, Shirley Stihler, Cynthia Jaynes, Hallie Morrow, Kay Ryan, Theresa Rossini, Gretchen Hester, Toni Gonzalez, Janet Canning, Ivette Pena, Linda Landry, Elissa Provance, Patric Widmann, Toni Doman, Robin Millar, Barbara Ferrera, Pat Winget, Sandy, Stephanie Pringle-Fox, Hedy Hansen, and Jean Brunelli for bringing me laughter and teamwork, Virginia Reynolds, and Sheila Wolfe, who labeled me the "Renaissance Lady," Nancy Sweet, Fran Chasen, Mary Lu Hickman, and Julie Jackson for believing in the power of touch. Last but not least, Suzie Stenseth and my valuable staff and friends at Community Therapies/Baby Steps, who keep on nurturing and nurturing even when you think there is no more to go around and who are always so supportive of anything I undertake.

This book could not have been written without the loving kindness of the many families who have participated in Dr. Elaine's TouchTime Baby Massage workshops. Some of the many parents and infants I can thank by name. For others who may not be listed, please know that I am eternally grateful and you are always in my heart. Thanks to: Beverly Shepard and Sumara; Darci and Desi; Desmond and Victoria; Eileen and Shea; Gabriela and Shaun Mack; Georgianna and Azijah; Jeanna, Brian, Cassidy, Leah, and Jacob; Jennifer and Matthew Horton; Jenny, Kevin, Summer Raine, Hailey, and Michelle Van Ornum; Joshua and Darren Martin; Karen and Michael Christy; Katie Clemm, Gary Dulak, Jan McCracken, and Sarah Jane and John Dulak; Linda Morgan and Melinda and Nita Loya; Lisa and Abigail Williams; Maria and Michael Leone; Mark and Ryder Rippel; Meredith and Bennett Fogel; Mitchell, William, and Ashton Frieder; Paula and Edgar; Rosa and Isac Acuna; Shannon, Robby, Stacey, and Michelle Santamaria; Sheri, Shawn, Jenna, and Corey Ebert and Michele Fogel; Sirah and Chance Henderson; Susan and Olivia Christina Stala; Susan, Yanir, Eliyah, and Liam Ram; Tara and Brayden Gheen; Zohar, Derek, Sarah, and Eliana McMurtry; and Margalit Ram.

There are so many others who have inspired me, supported me, and cared for me, and for those whom I may not have specifically mentioned, you know who you are, and I am forever grateful.

The time is yours. So find a comfortable chair and enjoy the information I am about to present to you. Feel your own energy. Sense your own mind/body connection. Then, with my love, I send you off to develop the first, most meaningful relationship that your baby will ever have, and that relationship is YOU!

Lovingly in touch,
Dr. Elaine

P.S.

A note about gender:

To avoid long and awkward phrasing within sentences, the publisher has chosen to alternate the use of male and female pronouns according to chapter. Therefore, when referring to your child, odd-numbered chapters use male pronouns, while even-numbered chapters employ female pronouns.

INTRODUCTION

What a wise decision you have made in selecting this book. Baby massage is a natural way to further brain development. Eye-to-eye contact enhances the development of the right side of the brain. Speaking to your infant during a massage assists in the development of the left side of the brain. Massage is a natural way of enhancing the physical and emotional well-being of your baby as well as providing increased intellectual performance. In addition, massage has been shown to increase gastrointestinal and metabolic efficiency, while promoting more active and alert babies who perform better on developmental tests than those infants who were not massaged. Furthermore, massage has been shown to have benefits for children who have arthritis, asthma, autistic tendencies, and for alleviating stress. Massage has also been shown to have benefits for those providing massage, too.

For everyone greeting an infant into his or her life, now or in the future, this book is written for you. Whether you are a biological parent, a surrogate parent, a foster parent, day care provider, or an extended family member, the word "parent" will be used interchangeably to mean "YOU." This book will show you an easy way you can develop a lifelong, loving connection with your baby that will lay the foundation for all of your child's future relationships.

The book begins with the most up-to-date research about the power of touch and the benefits of infant massage. In Chapter 1, I will explore with you the ways baby massage can have positive effects on your baby's brain development, as well as his or her physical and social-emotional well-being. I will share with you the importance of breath, energy, and the quality of your movements, and introduce you to the many hidden benefits that you will gain from baby massage, too.

Next, in Chapter 2, you'll be ready to begin, as I'll list the inexpensive, simple materials you can get to enhance your infant's massage. Guidelines are offered, which give permission to caregivers to perform the massage and remember the importance of bonding with their baby, whether in a full massage or an abbreviated massage. Massage oil ingredients are described, explaining the beneficial and harmful ingredients. When will you want to massage your baby? You will learn to observe the various states your baby goes through during the day, along with signs of your baby's willingness or unwillingness for massage.

After that, it's on to Chapter 3, and the basic stroke movements of Dr. Elaine's TouchTime Baby Massage. To make it simple and fun for you, I've turned these into ABCs: Attuning, Breathing, and Communicating. In fact, every stroke movement matches a letter in the alphabet to help you understand them and remember them. You'll see that massaging your baby is not a monologue, but rather a melodic interactive dialogue.

Once you are massaging, Chapter 4 shows how, during massage, songs and rhymes lead to added growth and development. Infant massage, when coupled with voice and rhythm, blends three languages: the language of touch, the language of words, and the language of melody. The songs and rhythms are another way of connecting with your baby, enriching communication moments, providing bonding and attachment, and improving relaxation for you and your baby.

Massage shouldn't end in infancy. In Chapter 5, we'll next talk about the benefits for your toddler, as well as techniques you may offer as you gain permission to begin the massage with him or her. I'll also give important tips for maintaining touch with older children and discuss the powerful benefits that are brought to both the child and the adult.

How do parents of a child with special needs ensure that they can massage their child without bringing harm? That's the next area we will tackle. In Chapter 6, parents will learn how to adapt to meet their child's needs. No matter what the special needs may be—autism, cerebral palsy, attention deficit hyperactive disorder, hypertonia, hypotonia, Down syndrome, cleft palate, or spina bifida—there are important ways massage can comfort and stimulate your child, while comforting and relaxing yourself and strengthening the relationship with your child.

Finally, we'll explore the exciting ways in which you are building a lifelong connection with your child. Guidelines will be given to ensure that the strokes of today mean plenty of success for decades to come.

Over the last thirty years, I have had the privilege of becoming one of the country's top infant massage experts and am called upon to speak, teach, and demonstrate nationally. My articles on the subject have appeared in both scientific and popular literature. I am even more privileged to be a parent of a loving college student and have seen firsthand, in my own family for many years, the results I describe in this book.

I am also privileged to hear the wonderful stories of other parents. I have heard a mother of a child with special needs say that before she began massaging him he was just "Patrick," and after the massage he had a personality all his own. I have heard a dad say that he didn't know how he would develop a bond with his child since he was gone so much of the time, but with massage they have developed a meaningful relationship and he now knows he has an important role in his son's life.

As these lucky parents discovered firsthand, the first language that your baby will experience in his or her life is not the language of words, but rather the language of touch. Whether that means being able to read your baby's cues, fostering communication, enhancing your baby's health, or creating loving and nurturing memories upon which your relationship will grow, with this book you are holding the map to it all in your hands. It is my intent that you will learn that within your hands, eyes, ears, voice, and heart, you hold the key to building a nurturing relationship with your child and facilitating a unique and special communication that will last a lifetime.

Just as I found my inner child while learning to become an infant massage instructor, I believe that through similar actions you will have the opportunity of rediscovering an ancient art that will provide you and your baby with hours of pleasure, while improving bodily functions and increasing your baby's brain development. You will sense the meaning of togetherness as your finger intertwines with the tiny finger of your baby, not knowing where your finger ends and your baby's finger begins. You will experience unity as your two breaths become one. You will sense the bond that connects and bridges the gap between you and your baby, and delight in the relationship that will last a lifetime.

CHAPTER 1

GROWING THE BODY— GROWING THE BRAIN

I remember back some twenty years ago, when my daughter was born, just like it was yesterday. Marveling at the miracle of her birth with my husband, I remember holding my daughter and breathing in her fresh new essence, feeling her soft new skin, and experiencing a fulfilling generational connection I had never felt before as a daughter or a sister, a wife or a friend. Now I was a mother. Now I was a parent. I held this tiny life in my hands and I held the universe and all the possibilities of who she would become. All the possibilities of how our life would be together as a family. I embraced the dreams of how she would grow, holding the dreams, hopes, and possibilities for humanity, as I held her in my arms and stroked her tiny five-pound, fourteen-ounce body.

It is just what the "doctor ordered" for both baby and parent when such soft, innocent, sweet, cuddly infants are created. Parents throughout the world desire only to hold their infants, love them, protect them, and nurture them. I knew from the moment I laid eyes on my daughter that I was in love with her, and her birth announcement proclaimed not only her name, her date of birth, weight and height statistics, but it also said "someone new to love."

There is no way that I could write a book about massaging your baby without sharing with all of you the power and magic of touch. Babies are born with seven senses (although five are most widely known). These are touch, hearing, sight, taste, smell, proprioception, and kinesthetics/movement sensations. (*Proprioception* detects the position of body parts in space and *kinesthetics* involves the vestibular system located in the middle ear that provides feedback about gravity, balance, and speed.) Touch is the first sense to appear in utero, and is central to the rest of our senses. Our other senses depend on touch for valuable information. When you hear your baby's cooing or babbling or crying, the three little bones in your inner ear are vibrating, touching one another, and sending your baby's message along the auditory nerve. Even while you are reading these words, perhaps unbeknownst to you, the air is touching your skin, registering temperature. Touch is a basic sense and yet one that has far-reaching importance for parents and babies alike.

In this chapter you will learn how baby massage offers you time to develop human connections and promote your baby's brain development. You will see how essential the sense of touch is for your baby's survival. You will discover the role touch plays in enriching communication, and forming secure attachments. Through massage, you will learn about the overall benefits of touch for you and your baby. You will also gain insight into how massage releases a natural dispensary housed within both of you that is open twenty-four hours a day, seven days a week. Landmark research studies will be shared that unequivocally show how absolutely vital massage and touch are for babies everywhere.

WHY USE TOUCH?

Touch is your baby's first means of communication.

Not only is touch the first sense that develops in the womb, but your baby's first experiences with the outside world are through the sense of touch. Whether it is moving down the birth canal, laying on the front of mommy's chest at the end of the birthing experience, or being held in daddy's arms after the umbilical cord is cut, your baby's first language of communication is through touch. We bond with our babies through touch. We relate to our babies through touch. We capture memories of love and compassion through touch.

Here is an acronym to contribute to your understanding of why touch is so vital for your baby and yourself. Spelled out to form the word CHEERS, it is my way of saying "Cheers" to all of you who are embarking on this miraculous baby massage journey.

Touch to Connect

For Baby: Your baby is developing trust and security in the first three months of life, making simple associations. Touching you, he connects to the most significant person in his world, experiencing the source of his own humanity and experiencing the closeness he felt in the womb. As you interact with your baby, nerve pathways are being made in your baby's brain at a remarkable rate of growth. Actually, if your baby's body grew at

DR. ELAINE'S TOUCH ACRONYM:		
CHEERS for your Baby and *CHEERS* for You!		
C	=	Connect and Communicate
H	=	Heal and Harmonize
E	=	Educate and Enable
E	=	Energize and Enhance
R	=	Regulate and Relax
S	=	Soothe and Socialize

a comparable rate of how much his brain grows, he could increase his weight from 8 pounds at birth to 165 pounds at one month old.

For You: It took nine months for your baby to arrive. You will form your own connections with your baby over time, which is known as bonding. You will also form attachments by holding your baby, kissing your baby, rubbing your baby, cuddling with your baby, and connecting skin to skin. Touching is an easy way for you and your baby to become related and relative to one another.

Touch to Communicate

For Baby: Touch was the first sense that developed in the womb. The message your baby receives is like a symphony of expression. He can sense your "touch-spoken" messages: "I am here for you. I will protect you and nurture you so much. Your needs are so important to me." Outside the womb your baby's reflexes communicate to you as he holds onto your finger, suckles at a breast, or gazes at you. If a picture is worth a thousand words, then a touch is worth a million!

For You: As a parent, you interact with your baby and the "communication dance" begins. By holding your baby, rocking your baby, and massaging your baby, you can communicate your feelings in ways that go deeper than words alone. While it has been stated that "in the beginning was the word and the word was with God and the word was God," we would not be here without touch. Touch is the primal language of communication.

Touch to Heal

Massage causes the "feel-good hormones" to be released throughout your baby's body, providing feelings of relaxation and well-being.

For Baby: All of your baby's systems—circulatory, digestive, respiratory, eliminative, nervous, muscular, immune, and endocrine—benefit from the ancient art of massage. Massage alters your baby's biochemistry. "Feel-good hormones" are released and the "fight, flight, and freeze hormones" are reduced during massage, healing your baby's body. Healing takes place as the immune system is strengthened and helps fight disease. When you are cuddling, hugging, and massaging your baby, you are actually causing the "feel-good hormones" to be released throughout your baby's little body, providing feelings of relaxation and well-being.

For You: Rubbing was a way that the ancient Greeks and those civilizations that came before them healed pains and injuries. It's amazing, but by massaging your baby, you will bring healing benefits to your own body. You will be able to lower your own blood pressure, slow down your own heart rate, and add relaxation to your own life. Massage heals the self at the body level, which further heals the self at a spiritual level, enlivening the connection with your baby that goes deeper than skin.

Touch to Harmonize

Through your unique touch signature—the shaping of your hands, rhythm of your strokes, gentleness of your touch—your baby identifies you from others.

For Baby: While you are massaging your baby, he experiences your rhythm, your voice, and your "touch signature." With the tempo of your touch and the quality of your hand shaping along your baby's skin, these rhythmic movements synchronize, bringing you closer together, blending, attuning, bonding, and attaching. This harmony goes beyond the visible. Even though our babies were created through touch, there are many other forces in the universe, like circadian rhythms, energy fields, and chemicals, that operate without being seen by the naked eye. For example, some studies have shown how baby massage may facilitate a baby's sleep pattern, which then matches the mother's pattern. Other studies reveal how some mothers who were depressed used massage and became less depressed, as did their babies.

For You: Have you ever listened to your own voice quality, or the voice patterns of others, when talking to babies? Usually a high-pitched, upward-inflecting voice pattern with short phrases is used. This is known as parentese. Once this pattern was labeled "motherese," but it recently became "parentese" to capture how both moms and dads change their tune while speaking with their babies. ("Cutchy cutchy coo." "Isn't that a

biiiig biiiig cat?" "Where's Alli-
son?" "I see you!" "Give daddy a
kiss . . . A big kiss!") You and your
baby develop a rhythm. Your
own "song." Your own "lyrics."
The harmony created with your
words and your touch grows the
body, brain, and emotions of your
baby, along with growing your
relationship.

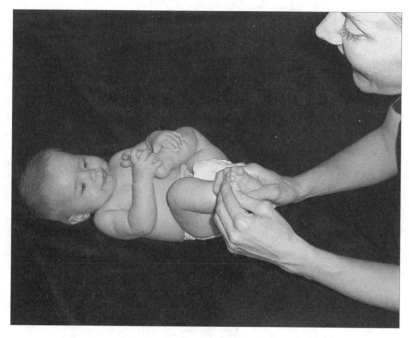

Touch to Educate:

For Baby: Your baby reaches out
with his hands, lips, and feet
to touch and feel things in his
world. This is the way he explores his world and learns about
sizes, tastes, temperatures, and
how things work. Babies have an abundance of touch-sensing organs in
their skin, which are more numerous in baby skin (up to three years old)
than in adult skin. Because of this enhanced sensitivity your baby will
experience touch far more intensively than you.

Babies enter the world
dressed in only their skin.
Through this largest bodily
organ and the sense of
touch they learn about
themselves and the world.

For You: You reach out and touch your baby. Just like your fingerprints are
unique, you have a special touch and a movement signature, which is also
unique. By using your touch patterns—the gentleness of your touch, the
shaping of your hands as you massage stroke by stroke, your movement
patterns, the rhythm of your strokes, the pacing of your massage, and your
voice patterns—your baby recognizes you from others and identifies you
as unique. You educate your baby about nurturing, trust, and caring
through your touch.

Touch to Enable

For Baby: You are assuring your baby's very existence and continuing his
very creation by touching him. Without touch your baby could not sur-
vive. Touch makes it possible for your baby to grow and improve his
mind, body, and emotions.

Your baby's brain will be pliable, growing dendrites and neurons from
the interactions he has with you. His brain becomes shaped by these social

Babies have an abundance of touch-sensing organs in their skin, which are five times greater in baby skin than in adult skin.

interactions, and the reciprocal give and take of a relationship through the basic primal sense of touch.

For You: Touch allows you the opportunity of getting closer with your baby to provide information in ways that are not always possible through words. Through your touch, you aid his learning about the world and you make possible the important secure attachment to grow your own relationship with your baby. Through your touch connection, you bring your baby the security and safety that he requires during the first year of life, which facilitate his learning and your own emotional satisfaction.

Touch to Energize

For Baby: Touch can be invigorating, increasing blood flow, relieving muscle aches and pains, and fostering more oxygenation to blood cells. The massage strokes can stimulate muscle tone, facilitating energy flow so that your baby's body will tap the source of energy from within.

For You: Massage reduces stress. When there is less stress, there is more energy available to your body. When I am stressed more than usual, I get a massage as soon as possible. I know that the massage will reduce my tension, and after the massage I will have renewed energy or a calmness that strengthens my overall psyche. Providing the massage, as you connect with your little one, you discover a flow of energy moving through you that you may not have known existed. This uplifting source of energy can invigorate you and alleviate stress.

Touch to Enhance

For Baby: Touch improves the quality of your parent-infant relationship. A soft embrace, a tender kiss, a caressing hand manifest as treasured actions memorized in your baby's psyche for a lifetime. Physiologically, your baby's bodily functions, respiration, elimination, circulation, and digestion are also enhanced. Your loving touch on his tummy and buttocks assists digestion and makes elimination easier. Emotionally, for a child, being understood and respected by a parent makes all the difference in the way he views himself and himself in the world.

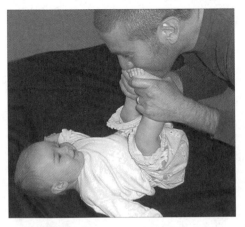

Daddy's kiss is a remembered treasure.

For You: Just as for your baby, massage will improve the

quality of your parent-infant relationship. You will sense a connection with your infant at a deeper level with secure attachment, understanding, and attunement. You will find the meeting place of your touch a place where you recognize and acknowledge your own contribution in the creation of your baby.

Touch to Regulate

For Baby: Like a valve that opens and closes the floodgates of emotions, different types of touch affect brain chemistry, releasing or reducing hormones throughout your baby's body and changing the way your baby feels and experiences day-to-day events. Nurturing touch will encourage your baby to be resilient, to "bounce back from frustration," and to self-regulate his emotions.

For You: Massaging your baby reduces or releases hormones in yourself. If you are a new mother, your baby's touch will release oxytocin, which facilitates the healing of your uterus after birth by contracting it, and your baby's touch will facilitate the release of prolactin, which furthers breast milk production.

> Massaging your baby reduces your blood pressure levels, calms your heart rate, and promotes relaxation.

Touch to Relax

For Baby: Massage leads to relaxation of tense muscles, deepening the release of melatonin, which improves your baby's sleep patterns, and increasing serotonin, which improves moods. So many feel-good hormones are released during the massage that many times you will find your baby falling asleep or getting very calm after you have massaged him.

For You: Massaging your baby leads to reducing blood pressure levels, calming your heart rate, reducing stress hormones, and promoting relaxation. Soon-to-be parents take my introductory workshop to find out about infant massage before they give birth. I always pass out plastic baby dolls so that they can experience some of the massage strokes they will use with their own baby. After a few strokes, when I look out at the audience of these soon-to-be parents with dolls on laps, I note their yawns and deep breathing. When I ask them

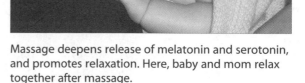

Massage deepens release of melatonin and serotonin, and promotes relaxation. Here, baby and mom relax together after massage.

about how they feel, they are always amazed that they could feel so relaxed by massaging just a plastic baby doll. I always tell them they will feel this way when their "real" baby arrives, too.

Touch to Soothe

For Baby: Remember when you hurt yourself and your mother or father hugged you or rubbed your knee or kissed your "boo-boo" to make it all better? Well, your baby is soothed by these acts of tenderness and kindness, and the additional pressure placed on his skin. Changing the energy field that was just disturbed by any hurtful action helps your baby return to a sense of balance.

For You: As a parent, you may get a sense that there is nothing you can do when your baby is crying from pain or discomfort. By touching your baby, comforting your baby, rubbing a hurt body part, or kissing the boo-boo, you find your way to reach out and ease your baby's hurt.

Touch to Socialize

For Baby: Humans are social beings. For each and every baby, massage provides a social connection, a time to bond with a significant caregiver. Within this social interaction, relationships are built and the brain is structured. Being touch deprived will result in retarded growth and malfunctioning of the body, brain, and psyche.

For You: The time you spend engaging in infant massage is time that allows you to become attached to your baby. This time facilitates the moments to use touch, speech, smell, and other senses while engaging in the social aspects of your species—eye gazing, smiling, and communicating. By massaging your own baby, it is as if you are touching the generations upon generations who have come before and those generations who will follow.

BIOLOGICAL NEED FOR TOUCH

Scientists have data that now supports what mothers of Eastern, Asian, African, European, Pacific Island, and other countries have passed down from generation to generation—touch and massage. You can see examples of touch in art and religious traditions. In Michelangelo's famous drawing on the ceiling of the Sistine Chapel, God's finger reaches towards Adam. In Christianity, Jesus intuitively knew and practiced the "laying on of hands" thousands of years ago.

The history of massage is long and without borders. As far back as 3000 BC, massage was practiced in China. There are records of the use of massage in India around 1800 BC. You can read about the importance of massage in the fifth century, when the famous Greek physician Hippocrates included massage in his days of treating and tending to the Greek people. When Emperor Frederick II attempted to study what would happen to children if they were raised without speech or cuddling in Germany in the year 1248, the children died before they could talk, and therefore he could not answer the question of his experiment.

When the Romanian orphanages were discovered and exposed in 1995, scenes of infants with developmental disabilities permeated the television screens, and news stories told about those who never survived. The infants who died had lacked touching, hugging, or cuddling. Others who had limited touch stimulation had developmental disabilities or were short in stature for their age. Some said that survival at the orphanage depended upon the location of the baby's crib. If the crib was close to the door and first in line for care, the child had a better chance for survival. If the crib was at the end of the line, he received little or no care and was apt to wither away and die, or suffer growth retardation.

Dr. Tiffany Field of the Touch Research Institute of Miami studied different citizens from cultures and countries around the world, and discovered that Americans touched less than the British did, who touched less than the French did. When Margaret Mead, noted anthropologist, went around the world exploring different tribes and people, she found that those people who were massaged during infancy were less aggressive and less violent. In American society today, many teachers are afraid to console a child who may have skinned a knee in the playground for fear of being accused of child abuse. There are also times that societies are confused about touch, so much so that parents may even fear touching their own children.

> Touch is a biological necessity.

However, touch is a biological necessity. Dr. Bruce Perry, Senior Fellow at the Child Trauma Academy in Houston, Texas, discovered that when touch and eye contact are absent, the frontal cortex of the brain does not grow. Touch cannot be considered an "add on" or a luxury—something one "spoils" a child with. Touch is necessary, just like the air we breathe, the water we drink, and the sunshine that nourishes us.

SCIENCE SUPPORTS WHAT INTUITION TELLS US

The pioneer work of Heidi Als and T. Berry Brazelton at Harvard; Tiffany Field and colleagues from the Touch Research Institute at the University of

Miami, Florida; Harry Harlow; Stephen Suomi; Marshall Klaus; John Kennell; Marian Diamond and Mark Rosenzweig at Berkeley; Saul Schanberg at Duke University; scientists at McGill University; and other researchers laid the foundation for massaging babies in the Western world. Some of their research studies used animal research. Other studies used infants and their mothers, or grandparents or other significant people in the babies' lives. They looked at the implications of touch and massage with babies in neonatal intensive care units or with babies displaying a variety of disorders or disabilities.

From the research experiments on animals, particularly rats, it was discovered that touch deprivation leads to growth retardation. From studies using monkeys, it was also discovered that contact touch, without nourishment, is more important than nourishment without contact touch. The hippocampus (part of the brain responsible for memory) seems to be more developed following a massage, and the immune system is also improved following touch.

Many of the studies using infants with special conditions have led to the current belief of the value of massage for all infants. It was surmised that if massage benefited those infants whose systems were so compromised at birth, imagine what massage would also do for babies who were born full-term with no complications.

WHY MASSAGE YOUR BABY?

Frederic Leboyer, an eminent physician and pioneer in birthing (1976) remarked that for a baby, massage was just as necessary as food. Using massage as a "two-way street," your baby learns about you as you learn about him! He learns about your touch signature—how your touch is different from others and what qualities make your touch different. How much pressure do you use? What speed is your stroke? What temperature are your hands? How do you shape your hands? What rhythm does your touch make on his body? How long do you take to breathe in between strokes? You learn how your baby likes to be massaged—what speed, what pressure, and even which body parts relax and calm your baby.

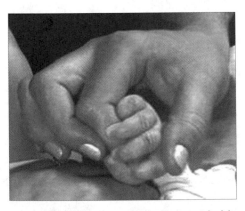
In these moments, it's indistinguishable where one finger starts and the other ends.

In these reciprocal massage moments, it is indistinguishable where one finger starts and the other body part ends, and in enjoying the time spent together, your energy and information merge. Your baby is memorizing the pleasure he shares with you massaging his legs, feet, arms, hands, chest, stomach, neck, back, or face. Your baby's body relaxes under your touch. He listens to your words. He watches your face smiling in the light. He hears a sweet lullaby. Learning takes place as your baby, in a quiet and alert state, welcomes exploration and feels secure.

As you massage your baby, you are creating an intimacy that will be able to span generations. Starting out as an infant, your baby grows into childhood, pre-adolescence, adolescence, adulthood, and parenthood. As a baby, he gives permission to receive a massage. As a child, he may verbally ask for a massage. As an adult, he remembers the gentle touch of his own parent, the communication and connection it enriched. As a parent, he has the chance to continue the cycle of massage. Now he will be able to offer a massage to his own baby. His baby will grow into childhood and adulthood and be able to ask for a massage. When he becomes a parent he will massage his own baby. As you become the aging adult, the family elder, your own children may seize the moment to offer you a massage. Massage becomes a family tradition that can continue through your children's children and reach future generations, as has been the case with many cultures of the world.

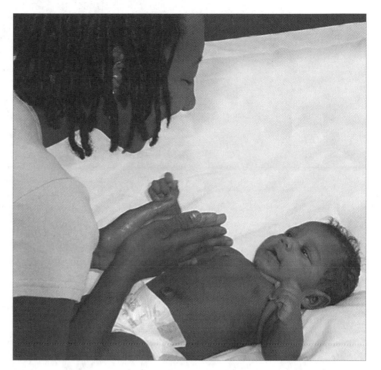

You're not just touching skin here, you are touching the miracle of life housed in the largest organ of the body—the skin. Touch your baby not just so he will touch you back, but so that he will touch his children and his children's children.

Staring into your baby's eyes, stroking gently and nurturing, you offer a connection to your baby that was once only realized as a fetus. In your embrace, you bring your baby close, as if to recreate the womb. You can fully experience the warmth, gentleness, and smoothness of your baby's soft skin, while your baby experiences the womb-like simulation of safety and security. Nowhere else will these memories be as strong as when you were touched by those who loved you and cared for you.

Learn About Each Other

As a parent, you want to do the best you possibly can to take care of your infant and meet his needs. In your busy, day-to-day hustle, infant massage allows you the opportunity to be in the moment with your baby, taking care of his needs while also taking care of your own needs. In these moments, you learn so many things about your baby (and yourself) that you may not have otherwise taken the time to learn. For example, by engaging in massage with your baby you will learn how to:

- Ask permission from your baby (talk to your baby before your baby is using words to talk to you), which respects your baby as an individual apart from yourself.

- Read your baby's body language (willingness or non-willingness to have a massage as described further in Chapter 2).

- Read your baby's bodily states, to determine whether your baby is in a quiet, alert state ready for a massage or not (see Chapter 2 for a listing of all of the body states).

Massaging the Pain Away

At twenty-six months of age, Edgar has neuro-fibro-matosis type I, a serious medical condition that causes him a lot of pain and suffering. When he wakes up in the morning from his sleep, he is in excruciating pain. Edgar's mom, Paula, learned baby massage to see if it would help ease his suffering. She would do anything to make his pain go away. To her surprise, the massages seemed to help. Edgar now asks his mother to rub his leg before he goes to bed, by pointing to his legs and saying "mommy hurt." Mom is more than happy to oblige his request.

When you massage your baby with your firm and gentle strokes, you are using the long nerves that send messages to the brain quickly; when the short nerves are massaged, the information takes longer to get to the brain. The "gate theory" developed by Melzack and Wall shows that there are long nerves and short nerves within our skin that go to the brain. Using the firm stroke in massage

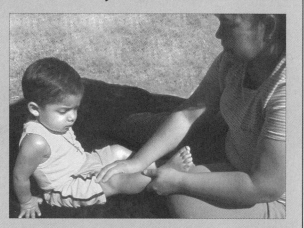

Any time is the right time for a massage. Just like the saying "Ask and ye shall receive," this toddler asked for and received a leg massage to ease his pain.

goes to the brain quicker and makes you feel better. This is also why having your mother "kiss your boo-boo" using her lips and putting pressure on the hurt always made you "feel better."

• Follow his lead, to determine which body part to massage and which one(s) not to massage.

• Read your baby's cues so that you can be a responsive parent and sensitive to his needs—traits needed to develop a secure and trusting relationship.

• Gain better understanding of your baby's likes and dislikes.

• Share reciprocal pleasurable moments together.

For yourself, by using baby massage, you can:

• Develop consistency with your baby.

• Establish routines with your baby.

• Learn how to create your own relaxation.

• Learn to set aside time to be together, which furthers bonding attachment, safety, security, and enjoyment.

• Gain confidence in your parenting skills.

• Gain competence in your parenting skills.

• Learn to go with the flow in parenting and massaging your baby. Become flexible and less rigid in how things "should look." So many parents become uptight when things don't go exactly as they had anticipated or how they think something should look. Massage allows you to "go with the flow." The strokes that your baby enjoyed and engaged in yesterday may not be the same ones he likes today. You realize that techniques are guides and not the "end all" or "be all." By reading your baby's cues, you may find you've altered your plans, while also deepening the understanding between both of you.

Bond and Form Secure Attachments

Being together with your baby affords you the opportunity to bond and further your attachment to each other. Noted child psychologists John Bowlby and Mary Ainsworth demonstrated the complexity and importance of infant attachment with a mother or primary caregiver, as secure attachment is a necessity for your baby to develop attention, to learn, and to build self-esteem. Using massage establishes an attachment relationship offering emotional connection and safety. Babies who experience this secu-

Dr. Elaine's Four Fundamental Pillars of CARE

Here are some ways that massaging your baby shows your infant how much you truly care, and fosters your child's secure attachment. Dr. Elaine's Four Fundamental Pillars of CARE for Supporting Bonding and Secure Attachment are: Consistency, Appreciation, Responsiveness, and Empathy. I believe they are all necessary to support your parent–infant attachment.

Dr. Elaine's Four Fundamental Pillars of CARE for Bonding and Connecting With Your Baby Through Massage

Consistency

- Set aside a time each day for massage or incorporate massage into daily routines. This can be done at bedtime each night, or when you change your baby's diaper, or during a special time of the day.

- Use a similar way to begin every massage. You can ask the same question each time you start, such as "Are you ready for a massage?" You can warm the oil in your hands by swishing your hands near your baby's ear, or hold up your hands for your baby to see the oil.

- Utilize your own "touch signature" made up of your unique rhythm, breath, movement quality, speed, and pressure, which becomes the way your baby knows it's you who is holding him, stroking him, and massaging him. This will develop over time.

- Use similar strokes for each body part, gliding, pressing, rubbing, circling, fanning, and rolling.

Appreciation

- Recognize the "heartthrob" your baby is to you. My husband would say that being with our daughter would "make his spine tingle." Some of the massage strokes include names to instill this special feeling, such as "dear heart," "dear one," and "divine prayer."

- Attune with your baby. In the moment of massage you are in unison, reading cues and harmonizing with one another, adjusting to the different movements of your baby.

- Accept your baby for who he is. Be in the moment with your baby: breath in and out together, connecting to one another through touch.

rity in loving relationships may be able to face adversity with more adaptability. Some examples are when your baby is able to adapt to mother's consoling arms when his favorite "blankie" is put in the washing machine to be washed, or when the little rattle he loves to play with is taken to his cousin's house by mistake. Dad can replace the rattle with his set of car keys and his comforting touch.

Alan Stroufe and his colleagues present strong evidence of the link between early care and a child's later capacity to connect with others. It is so essential to the development of attachment behavior and early social development of your young child that both you and he have the capacity to elicit and respond to behaviors in mutually pleasurable ways.

- Appreciate the miracle of life before you and the wonder your baby brings.
- Appreciate the magnificence of the human body and how, through massage, you are able to release and reduce hormones creating a healthier, happier, and more relaxed child and self.

Responsiveness

- Watch your baby's reactions while you massage, and change a stroke or a position if your baby indicates the need to do so.
- Stop the massage and provide a "cuddle break" or attend to basic needs (hunger, pain, diaper change, etc.), if and when needed.
- Be flexible with each massage. Don't expect each massage to be exactly the same.
- Let your baby know that you are listening to him and responding to his needs.

Empathy

- Be sensitive to your baby's cues: facial gestures, body language, emotional states including noticing your baby's quiet alert state (see Chapter 2 for more information), which is the preferred state for massage.

- Listen to your baby's story as he "vents" while you massage different body parts (chest, stomach).
- Figure out what each cry, grimace, whimper, or babble means.
- Feel your baby's experience. Sense the significance of your baby's first three years and all the learning and brain development that is taking place daily.

I remember when twins Sarah Jane and John were receiving one of their very first massages. Their parents were massaging their faces and used the CARE approach. Consistency: They first massaged their baby's temples, and moved to their sinuses and then to their lips. Appreciation: No sooner were the twins' lips massaged did they begin to pucker, and move their lips as if remembering the sucking sensation of drinking. Responsiveness: Their massages came to a temporary halt as both began crying. Mom made milk available to them as they began to suckle on the nipple placed inside their mouths. Empathy: The sense of touch had triggered their nipple request and their empathetic mom answered their cries with the nourishment they sought. When you use CARE in massaging your baby, your baby will feel SAFE (SAFE stands for secure *attachments* for *everyone*.)

Dr. Bruce Perry found that a majority of attachment problems comes not necessarily from parental abuse, but rather from parental ignorance of how to provide optimal care during early childhood. He found that one out of three infants have impaired attachment with their primary caregiver, which results in difficulty in intimate relationships and requires years of psychotherapy to undo the damage caused during a few crucial months in early childhood.

By instructing parents in massage, I have seen them develop secure relationships with their infants and children, in ways that they can easily grasp. When I appeared on The Learning Channel's *A Slice of Life*, a mom and her son, Connie and Caleb, appeared with me. Caleb was Connie's first son and had been born prematurely. I had instructed her in Dr. Elaine's TouchTime Baby Massage. This is what Connie said:

> Elaine has taught me to do things with Caleb that I haven't been able to do before. Just calming him down through the massage techniques, and (having) playtime . . . with mommy. We bonded together so much with the massage technique.

Another parent, Felicia, who is a child development specialist at Baby Steps early intervention program, said:

> When I massage my child I know I make my child feel good, and feel comfortable. He experiences my love and he knows and understands that through touch we can communicate. With our bonding and attachment we will be close for the rest of our lives.

Your babies are precious gifts and secure attachments will ensure resiliency in their daily lives, which means that they will be able to tolerate high intensity emotional states—loss of loved ones, changed plans, broken promises, and other numerous challenges.

Build Baby's First Relationship and Shape Neural and Body/Mind Connections

Your baby's basic needs are to feel loved and to have a sense of belonging. Everyone, babies and adults included, have a basic need to connect with other human beings. We are our baby's very first relationship. Through massage we also discover a way to facilitate our baby's first relationship. Massage does not just stroke skin. With two willing people, baby and you, massage opens a dialogue to build trust, security, health, happiness, and relaxation, while "penetrating into the core of one's being."

Through massage, you enrich your baby's physical development (muscle tone, weight gain, increased sleep); physiological development (circulation, digestion, respiration); intellectual development (memory and attention); and social-emotional development (friendliness, secure attachment, and self-regulation). This lays the foundation for all future relationships to follow.

Relationships not only influence brain development. According to Dr. Daniel Siegel, educator, psychiatrist, and award-winning author of *The Developing Mind* (1999), relationships "structure brain growth."

When your baby is born, many of his organs are miniature organs. As

Touch is absolutely necessary for your baby's brain development.

your baby grows, so do those body parts! Let's take for example your baby's heart. It has all of the necessary parts to pump blood through your baby's body. As your baby gains weight and grows longer, your baby's heart will get bigger and continue pumping with greater ferocity, pushing blood through the body and oxygenating the blood that is returned to it from your baby's veins. But not all body parts are in this miniature state. Other parts require more nurturing for them to develop.

The brain is one organ that doesn't follow the growth pattern of the heart. Coming through the birth canal at nine months of age is a good thing because your baby wouldn't be able to get through the birth canal if he stayed in the womb much longer. His head would be just too big! But as Ashley Montague stated, in his seminal book *Touching: The Significance of the Skin,* you now have a baby who's growing his brain *outside* of the womb after spending nine months of growing it inside the womb!

Is there a problem if the brain is still growing outside the womb? How long do we have to cultivate this brain growth and who is responsible for growing your baby's brain? Touching and infant massage (as part of your baby's environment) provide the nurturing that is needed for developing your baby's brain, while your own genetic make-up provides the nature that was needed to develop your baby in the first place.

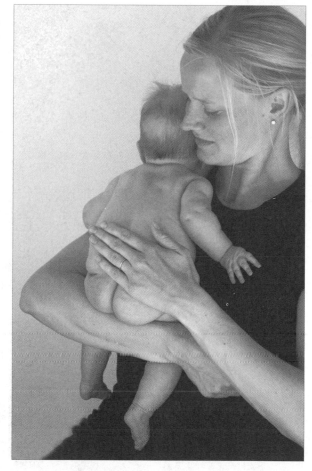

Nurturing your baby through touch, you stimulate and regulate your baby's natural pharmacy, which maximizes health and well-being.

Your baby's brain grows by how you nurture him. Physicians can spend days and days talking about whether feeding breast milk or formula to your baby is best, but one of the simplest ways to "feed" your baby is through touch. This is how infants have been fed since the beginning of time. No matter what nationality or culture, babies usually arrive through the birth canal (unless Cesarean section is necessary), and are held, stroked, caressed, rubbed, hugged, patted, cuddled, and fondled.

Through touch, the primal communicator, your baby's brain grows. When your baby is born, his brain weighs about twelve ounces. His brain will double in weight by the time he is one, and by five years of age he will have a brain that will be about 90 percent of its adult weight of almost three pounds. Your newborn's billions of neurons will make 1,000 trillion synaptic connections and dendrite connections between nerve cells, and, within the brain, will either grow and organize (with the information that your baby receives) or, like a tree, be pruned if not needed. Touching your baby is not only a pleasurable experience for both of you—touching your baby is a way of nurturing your baby that is absolutely necessary for your baby's brain development. You must nurturingly touch your baby for your baby to grow. As Dr. Candace B. Pert, noted neuroscientist, stated in *Molecules of Emotions* (1999), "the body is the gateway to the mind." As you touch your baby, you are stimulating and regulating your baby's natural pharmacy at "precisely the right time in exactly the appropriate dosages to maximize feelings of health and well-being."

Let's look at little Karl, who was born full-term. His mother and father were thoroughly overjoyed to have their baby arrive. In the hospital after his birth, he was placed on his mother's tummy and, moving upward and suckling at her breast, helped mom produce prolactin, enabling more milk production. Karl was also allowed to fall asleep on his mommy's chest, which allowed him to regulate his heartbeat and his temperature. Sucking strongly at his mother's breast allowed the chemical oxytocin to flow, which then assisted in contracting mom's uterus. Maria held her son, as did her husband Juan, and continued talking to him and stroked him ever so gently at first, structuring his brain. As Maria held him in a soft warm blanket with a little more pressure, it was as if she was returning him to her womb. Mom and dad were feeling content. Karl was feeling content and secure. The world was in their hands, just as the world had been in mine, when my daughter was born.

What may not be visible to the naked eye, but is visible by magnetic resonance imaging equipment, is that as Karl's parents stroke him, Karl's brain is growing dendrites. As his parents hold him, touch him, and fall in love with him, he is growing the right side of his brain. As his par-

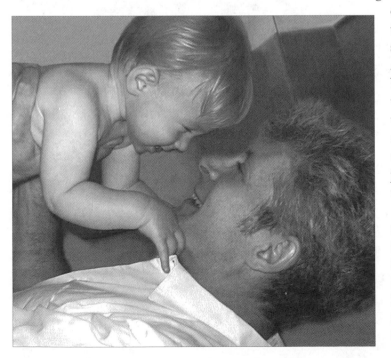

Through touch this baby is learning, and growing his brain and emotional intelligence within a loving parent-infant relationship.

ents speak to him and explain to him how happy they are to see him, he is growing the left side of his brain. Simultaneously, touch is maximizing Karl's feelings of health and well-being and releasing his emotions. As his family continually responds to his needs and comforts him, Karl is learning about the security and safety of his world. This might not be the typical scene of what you might have in mind for learning to take place. You may think that your child has to be watching an educational tape, or listening to Mozart CDs, or playing with an object, for his brain to be growing. But now you know that through the power of touch, in the context of a relationship, your child is growing neural connections uniting his body and mind, without the need of a costly toy or object.

Siegel eloquently stated that the mind emerges from the neural connections that have been shaped by human connections. He further affirms that the brain's function and structure are directly shaped by "interactions with the environment, especially relationships with other people." This concept is a major shift in thinking, for now as you are massaging your baby, you are actually shaping the development of his brain structure, along with unleashing pleasurable hormones and neuropeptides located throughout your baby's body (and your own). As both you and your baby reciprocally interact with one another, the body and mind can not be separated. The relationship that is forming will structure his brain and his emotions.

The importance of relationships in your infant's life cannot be underestimated. The first three years of life are critical in the development of your baby's brain, and the first relationship your baby has is with you, his primary caregiver, and it lays the foundation for all future relationships. The days of nature vs. nurture are gone, and now we look at nature and nurture as important partners for your baby's growth. It is human nature to be touched. It is nurturing touch that will create safe and trusting relationships. You, as the center of your baby's universe, have the potential of nurturing your baby to his fullest potential.

HOW MASSAGE MERGES PROCESSES OF GROWTH

Although books and scientific papers separate touch as a sense, truly there can be no separation among the senses. All systems and senses including biological, intellectual, and socio-emotional processes work together. Whether you massage your little baby at four weeks of age, after his umbilical cord ending has fallen off, or at four months of age, aside from building relationships and structuring your baby's brain, massage enlivens hearing, seeing, feeling, tasting, movement sensation, and balance.

Imagine massaging your baby, totally attuned, while your baby is looking back at you. If he could talk he might say, "I smell your sweet fragrance. I hear the harmonic sounds of a lullaby. I see your smile and I sense the tender and firm pressure of your hands along my leg using massage oil. I sense the rhythm of your movements in tune with me and feel the shaping of our bodies moving our breath in and out. I am so in love with you, and feel so close and connected. My heart is beating with yours and I feel calm, happy, and secure."

Think about your own childhood. Are there any people you remember even now for the kind of hug they gave you, or the way they held you, or the way they kissed you, or when they massaged you? One family member I can remember with glee is my jovial Great Uncle Charlie with his handlebar moustache, his hearty laugh, his fragrant cologne, and the biggest hug you could ever get that went clear around my whole body. That memory of his touch, his voice, his cologne takes me back at least forty years. How far back does your memory take you? Will you be the individual who invokes such memories for your little one when he is mature?

BENEFITS FOR DADS, TOO

Dads interact with their babies differently than moms—check out this football hold!

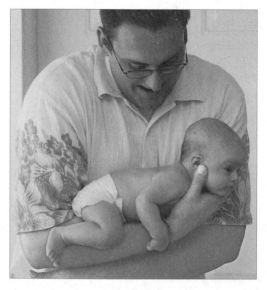

I wanted to make this section separate because so many times when dads read this type of book about massaging your baby, they may not see themselves doing the massaging. A dad may have a fear of "breaking his baby" because his hands are so big and usually one hand can cover the entire back of his newborn. Or when your baby gets a little older and may not be talking yet, as a dad, you may feel that there is nothing much that you can even say.

I remember Jerry, who had just had a son, but felt that since his son couldn't speak yet, or throw a football, that he wouldn't have much to do with him until he was older. He was unsure of his role with his baby, and didn't know how he could spend any nurturing time with him until he grew up a bit. Then there was Josh, a first-time dad who picked his son Darren up in his arms from the time Darren was born and held him like a football. Then he held him like an airplane, and then kissed and hugged him, talking to him all the time. Josh realized that he could play an important part in his son's life from birth, different from the role that his wife would play, but equally important.

No matter which parent you are, you will have your very own "touch signature," and your child will benefit greatly from experiencing different signatures from each parent. What was once regarded as a husband's role to support his wife during pregnancy and after is now seen a bit differently, as dads are taking more active roles in their baby's growth and development.

Your wife had your baby inside her womb for nine months. She can breastfeed your baby, which creates an immediate body intimacy that you cannot provide. Even though you may have felt your wife's pain, you will never know how it felt to carry a baby inside yourself for nine months, sleeping with a pillow between your legs because of the discomfort, or breathing so hard that you didn't think the baby would ever come.

When you learn the joy of TouchTime Baby Massage, however, you bridge the distance between your infant and yourself. You can learn to read your baby's cues: facial expressions and body language. Reading your baby's cues helps you to get to know your baby more intimately. Learning about the different effort-shape qualities of touch can also assist you in lessening any fears you may have about your own strength in comparison to your baby's. Rhythm, temperature, pressure, speed, direction of strokes, and the shaping of your hands are all aspects of massage that you can learn if you are willing. Using your breath will also help you relax with your baby.

Learning baby massage can alleviate the feeling of being left out, and not knowing how to bond. Susan told me that her husband, loving and supportive as ever, "scored additional points" with her when he learned TouchTime Baby Massage. Yanir gave Susan the gift of a "shower break"—the one necessity that almost becomes a luxury for a mom once her baby is born. If you, the dad, learn baby massage, your wife can luxuriate for five, ten, or fifteen minutes in the shower while you enjoy the luxury of being warmed by the touch of your own baby holding your hands, looking up at you, and learning your daddy "touch signature." Being in rhythm through touch allows you to harmonize and synchronize with one another. Being together and responsive to your baby establishes a genuine relationship as you grow the structure of your baby's brain. Massaging your baby brings "cheers" to both you and your baby (as stated earlier in this chapter), and has lifetime effects on learning and growing for both you and your baby.

Now that you know about the miracle of touch and the importance of massaging your baby, and you understand that when you are massaging your baby both you and your baby benefit, it's time to find out what it takes to prepare for massaging your baby. Some of you may wonder how long it will take to learn the techniques. Others may wonder if you will ever have time to fit massage into your busy day. Others may be ready and willing to give massage a try. No matter which category you fit into, rest assured that by reading this first chapter, you have gained a strong massage foundation. All you need to learn now are the steps for getting ready. It's as easy as 1–2–3. So let the preparation begin!

Chapter 2

GETTING READY

You might think that unless your baby is crying or "throwing a fit" your baby is ready for a massage. You'd be surprised to know that there is more to learn about baby massage than that! This chapter will provide checklists and charts to enhance your knowledge about the seven simple do's and don'ts of baby massage, different behavioral states your baby goes through daily, and which is the optimal state for massage. You will also learn what you need to prepare for the massage, and reasons why you may not want to massage your baby (contraindications).

You will see how easy and natural it is to massage your baby, especially when your baby and you are willing. No matter what time of the day—morning, afternoon, or night—anytime is the right time when there are two willing people and contraindications have been ruled out.

Let your rhythm flow, from your touch to your baby's skin. Let your energy fill your baby with tender loving care that only you can bring, and let sweet smiles and giggles and coos tell you how much your baby is enjoying the time you are spending together. Massaging your baby will establish lasting memories for your baby and yourself, increasing health and happiness as you experience your baby's uniqueness, each skin fold, each dimple, and the relaxation and joy massage brings to both of you.

RECOGNIZING YOUR BABY'S ENERGY LEVELS

Babies are people, too, cycling through various behavioral states day or night. Within twenty-four hours, you may see your baby quiet and drowsy, transition to an alert state, and become uncontrollable as she cries at the top of her lungs. Just as babies move through these cycles throughout the day, sometimes more abruptly than others, they may move

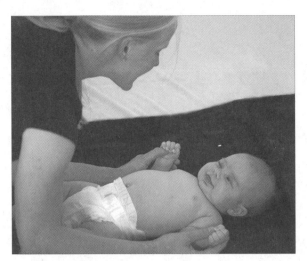

Baby is all smiles in her quiet alert state as she takes in her world, with mom present and attuned with her baby.

Mom is all smiles as her baby sleeps peacefully after his massage.

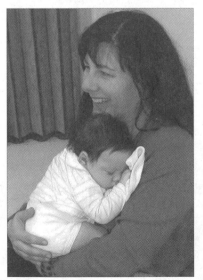

through these cycles during the massage you offer. Don't be surprised by the changes you will see. Simply recognize change as a natural course of events in the life of your infant.

For a massage, the optimum attuning state for your baby to be in is the state of *quiet alertness*. In this state your baby is open to receiving you and engaging with you as she smiles, possibly babbling, with her eyes open and alert. She is not moving too actively or squirming. She is quietly alert, taking in the world, with you in it!

I am reminded of little Michael, only two months old, who started out in a quiet alert state, moved into the crying state, moved back into the quiet alert state, and then ended in the deep sleep cycle. His mother, Maria, experienced his behavioral changes and learned so much about her son. As Michael learned to trust his mother and feel secure in her arms, Maria learned to trust her parenting skills and allow her son his time moving in and out of these cycles, as she comforted him, responding sensitively to his needs, deepening the give and take of their relationship, and thereby deepening their bond.

On page 29 are some descriptions of the seven behavioral states, so that you will be able to recognize each state and know the best time for giving your baby a massage.

RECOGNIZING YOUR FEELINGS, TOO

We can see how important it is to recognize the state your baby is in prior to the massage, so that you can read her cues. Now let's explore what you are telling your baby when you offer her a massage. Why should you care about how you feel when you offer a massage, especially since you know that the massage will relax you and your baby? Well, relaxation may be the end product, but what about the journey? The simple explanation is your baby can feel your energy! If you think you must give a massage before you leave the house to go food shopping, or you are worried that you won't have time to get a full massage in before your baby gets too active, then the quality of the massage and the benefits to you and your baby will be compromised. Here are some clues for you to determine when you should give your baby a massage:

Stages of Waking and Sleeping	What Baby May Be Saying
DEEP SLEEP	**"Don't wake me! I am so deeply asleep."** I don't even hear you, and will not respond to a lullaby or nursery rhyme.
QUIET SLEEP	**"Let me be!"** I am sleeping, and moving ever so slightly. You can see my breathing changing.
LIGHT SLEEP	**"Just a little longer."** You may think I am getting up, but I am still sleeping. My eyelids may be fluttering, and you may hear me making some sounds as I sigh, but I am still sleeping ever so lightly.
DROWSY	**"Not yet!"** I am getting up, ever so slowly. I may have a "dazed" look about me with my eyes partly opening. I am moving and making sounds.
QUIET ALERT	**"Yes! Yes! Yes!"** This is the best time for my massage. I am wide awake. My eyes are open and I am ready to engage with you. Let's communicate.
ACTIVE ALERT	**"Playtime!"** I won't lie still enough for a massage. My arms are thrashing about, and so many colors and objects capture my attention.
CRYING	**"No way!"** I am fussy and irritable and cannot attend to anything right now. Perhaps after I am comforted I will be ready for our massage or to continue the massage we had started.

Don't provide massage with your baby when you are:	Provide massage with your baby when you are:
Tired	Alert
Upset	Happy
Agitated	Calm
Sick	Vibrant
Angry	Pleasant
Stressed	Relaxed

Even if you know how vital massage is for the well-being of your baby and yourself, for both your sakes don't provide massage when you are tired, upset, agitated, sick, angry, or stressed—as your baby will feel your energy and the time you spend together will not be attuned or engaging in a positive way. It is difficult to read your baby's cues and follow your baby's lead when you are consumed with your own agitation or anger. It would be best to wait until you are more relaxed, happy, calm, vibrant, and feeling stress-free.

I am reminded of Erica, a lovely young woman, who was looking forward to baby massage with her newborn daughter, Julia. She couldn't wait for four to six weeks to come so she could give her daughter, Julia, her first massage. Erica knew how important this time together would be for her daughter's growth and development and for their parent-infant bonding. Erica visualized and thought about this first massage for weeks and weeks. She really wanted their first massage to be perfect. When the day that Erica had been dreaming about finally came, she gave her neck a deep rotation, remembered to ask Julia's permission, which she received, and began the massage stroke of stroking her daughter's little leg. She began massaging from the hip down to the foot. But Julia cried and cried and Erica could not console her, until all that Erica could do was stop stroking her, pick her up, and attempt to soothe her (usually amicable) daughter.

When I questioned Erica several days later about what she thought had happened with her experience with Julia that day (she was too upset after this experience to describe her feelings that same day), she told me how nervous she had been about getting it right! Erica's own worry and her desire for perfection translated into a nervousness that was felt by Julia, which altered Julia's behavioral state. Julia, usually an agreeable baby, turned into a fussy one that day. From a quiet alert state she went into a crying state.

Once Erica realized how much pressure she was putting on herself to provide a perfect massage and get everything right, she realized that she would have to let it go and be in the moment of the massage, mutually sharing the time together with Julia. Subsequent massages were easier and enjoyable for both Erica and Julia.

It is essential that you are relaxed when you give your baby a massage.

Erica learned about her own stress levels and how to relax herself before starting to offer a massage to Julia. Erica also learned that when she has less time than she would like, she offers Julia a brief massage, of possibly only one body part, and ends the massage with an easy back rub. Erica is more comfortable knowing that massage is less about strokes, and more about being together with her baby while sharing special moments united through touch.

Erica and Julia now engage in massage time on a regular basis and Erica is aware of her own body states. She relaxes herself before beginning and doesn't worry about getting it right, or giving the perfect massage. Through massage, she realized that most of the time she had been stressed out about getting "parenting right" and now she realizes she is the "right parent." She remembers to breathe more throughout the day, which translates into a more relaxed parent and a more relaxed baby.

Erica's experience with baby massage was quite different from Mitchell's massage with his son William. Every time Mitchell finished his massage, he didn't know who was more relaxed—his son or himself. He didn't have a picture in his mind of what the massage should be. Rather, he and William captured the moment and experienced the rewards of the give and take of their communication through touch.

INTERPRETING YOUR BABY'S CUES

Your baby is speaking to you long before she uses words. Interpreting your baby's cues is one of the most important parenting skills you will learn through baby massage. Your baby will develop trust and security when you show sensitivity to her needs. By observing her body language, and learning the meaning of her actions, including cries, you will begin to understand your baby's wishes and desires.

You may be able to tell when your baby is anxious or tired or hungry. You may watch your baby go into a "fussy" state and wonder if she has an upset stomach or needs a diaper change. By watching and listening to your baby, you begin to know your baby's habits. For instance, you may wonder why your baby is crying during a massage.

Eight Reasons for Crying During Baby Massage

Your baby may be saying:

❏ "I'm too hot or too cold. My clothing needs to be taken off or put on."

❏ "I'm dirty. Change my diaper."

❏ "I'm hungry. Feed me."

❏ "I'm feeling ill."

❏ "I want to be picked up and held."

❏ "I've had enough. It's time to stop."

❏ "I need a change."

❏ "I have something to say and want you to listen."

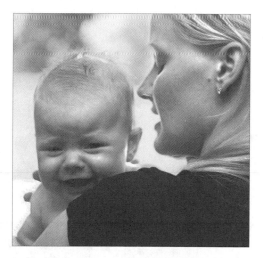

Your baby cries for many different reasons. What do you think this baby's crying is saying?

Even if your baby is in a quiet alert state, this isn't a 100-percent guarantee that she will accept your inquiry, "Do you want a massage?" This vital question must be asked before any infant massage begins.

By knowing which cues mean "I'm ready" and which cues mean "No, not now," you gain great strides in growing your relationship. By knowing which cues mean that your baby is "available" for engaging with you in a massage, and which cues mean that your baby is "unavailable," it

Interpreting your baby's cues is one of the most important parenting skills you will learn through baby massage.

nurtures your parent-child bond by respecting your child's state of being and respectfully seeing your baby as a unique individual. This sensitivity helps your baby feel acknowledged and understood, and allows you the opportunity to meet the social and emotional needs of your infant. Also, this allows your baby the opportunity to know that you are respecting your time together during the massage.

The time together will be best spent when *both* your baby and you are ready and willing. By making sense out of your baby's cues and understanding her feelings, your baby is feeling cared for and understood, learning that it is okay to express feelings, and beginning to understand how others feel. Your baby is feeling empathy and understanding from you, which leads to helping your baby develop trust, security, and emotional regulation.

In *Promoting First Relationships* (2003), Kelly, Auckerman, Sandoval, and Buehlman describe a path to trust and security that includes many of the same elements of infant massage. Some of these elements include your close physical contact; listening and responding to baby's sounds as you gaze into her eyes; watching cues; gently holding and rocking your baby; and describing how your baby feels. Gently singing or rhyming; being responsive and consistent in how you care for your baby while honoring natural rhythms; using loving rituals; and having fun on your baby's level also contribute to establishing a safe and nurturing world for your baby.

Mom is joyfully present and available, watching her baby's cues to determine the next massage stroke movements.

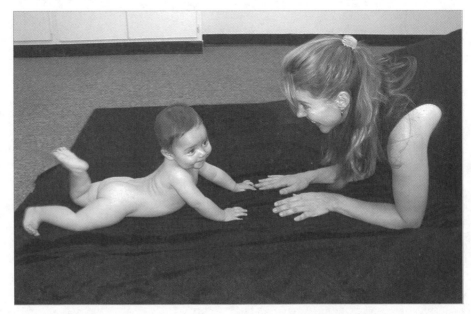

DETERMINING YOUR BABY'S READINESS

Let's find out about the different cues that your baby may give you to help you know whether she is, or is not, in the mood for a massage. In technical terms, these are called *engagement* and *disengagement* cues or, this is when your baby is saying "Yes, I am ready for a massage," or "No, I don't want one now!" Your baby may alternate between these signals, so that although she may have told you that she had enough, by reading that cue and then by comforting her—perhaps holding her up so she can see the world over your shoulder—she may then be ready to engage in the massage again.

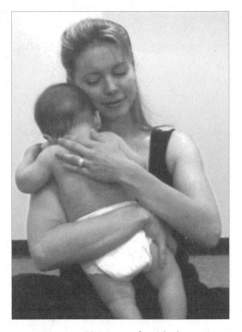

I am reminded of Chance, a little boy who began squirming with every stroke that his mother Sirah gave him. She then decided to lift him up and hold him in her arms, talking to him and patting him on his back. When she was finished with that three-minute exchange, he looked into her eyes, she calmly put him back down on the cushion, and he allowed her to massage the rest of his leg, which before he had not wanted her to touch.

Your baby is saying "yes" or "no" using a variety of body language, sounds, and gestures. Here are some of the cues you can read to know whether your baby wants to continue or discontinue the massage:

Mom comforts baby, providing a special "hug break" until baby is ready to resume his massage.

Engagement Cues **"YES, I AM READY!"**	*Disengagement Cues* **"NO, NOT NOW!"**
Baby is looking at you	Baby turns eyes away
Baby is smiling	Baby is frowning or making a face at you
Baby's arms and legs are quiet	Baby's arms and legs are squirming, flailing, kicking
Baby is holding your arm, reaching out	Baby is batting you
Baby's eyes are wide and bright	Baby's eyes are dazed and dull
Baby is cooing, babbling, conversing	Baby is crying
Baby puts hand to mouth	Baby arches back
Baby is calm	Baby is hiccupping, spitting up, vomiting, or wrinkling forehead

Following Your Baby's Lead

Remember, with baby massage you are following your baby's lead. Although you think you have the ideal plan to begin the massage at a certain body part and end with a back massage, your baby may take you on another course. You must become a reader of your baby's cues, and have the flexibility to allow the massage to move from one body part to another based on the messages your baby sends you.

For example, Adrienne and her son Marcus started the massage attuning interactively with one another. Adrienne got close to her baby as she sat in a comfortable position, relaxed her neck muscles, and inhaled and exhaled while rotating her head. Marcus was in a quiet alert state and ready for engagement. Attuning with Marcus, Adrienne calmly placed her hands near his ears, rubbing her palms together with natural baby massage oil. Marcus's wide-open eyes and quiet and alert body told Adrienne very clearly that he was ready for a massage. After enjoying the massage of his right leg, Marcus appeared ready for massaging his right foot. Using observation, thereby reading his cues, Adrienne saw that Marcus was displaying discomfort, withdrawing his foot away from her, and flailing his arms. So rather than continue to massage the right foot that gave him discomfort, she began holding his right foot in her loving hand, telling him how much she loved him.

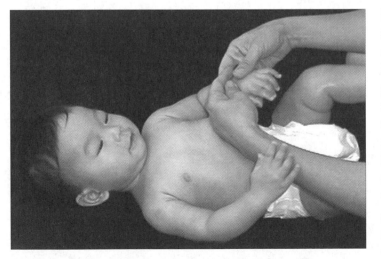

This little one is smiling at his mom, with quiet legs and one hand reaching out to mom's arm, as if to say, "Keep massaging, this feels so good." Happily his mom follows his lead.

Adrienne felt Marcus release his foot as she simply held it. Her son then allowed her to massage his foot. Adrienne had understood his cue, pacing her movement to align with his cues, giving Marcus the opportunity to relax. If he had not released his foot and was still not ready to proceed with a massage of that body part, she could have checked to see if he was ready for massaging another body part. If he were not agreeable, then she would let go of that desire to massage his foot, and realize that there would be another opportunity—when both are willing to engage in massage together.

Just like Marcus, throughout the day and during the massage, your baby will be giving you a variety of signals. She may turn away from you, indicating that she has had enough. Then, as you pause and stop stroking, she may turn back towards you and signal that she is ready again. Your watchful eyes, listening ears, and loving heart will be able to read her cues and determine if the massage can continue. Other times, your baby's signal may be an unwilling cue that will end the massage for that time period, as she may need to have her diaper changed or have a cuddle break, or as she begins kicking, squirming, and turning away from you, which signals that she has had enough for now and needs some time to self-regulate.

I am reminded of Connie, (you met her and Caleb in Chapter 1,) who read her son Caleb's cues. He became "fussy" when she was massaging his stomach. She sensed that he wanted to be held rather than continue with massage. She stopped the massage, picked him up, and said in a loving voice, "Do you want a hug now?" Connie gently hugged him, allowing him a position change. She held him in her arms, talking to him and gently patting him on his back. When mom was finished with that exchange, Caleb looked into his mother's eyes. Connie calmly put Caleb back down on the soft blanket and he allowed her to massage the rest of his stomach. In his own time, he had become ready again. Connie was successful in reading her son's return to quiet alertness, and by putting him back on the massage mat and getting permission ("Do you want to continue? Are you ready now?"), Caleb answered back with wide-open eyes, calmly and happily smiling back to her.

Just like these two examples of baby massage with Marcus and Caleb, remember, you are following your baby's lead. Even though Adrienne and Connie may have had an ideal plan when engaged in massage, their babies took them on another course of action. They read their babies' cues, and had the flexibility of changing their baby massage sequences when the boys directed them. Being flexible and reading cues will actually allow you to gain confidence in your parenting. As your baby responds to your back-and-forth interaction, you will get to know your baby's desires and needs. This is the way you connect as a parent.

Listening With Your Ears and Heart

Whatever your baby's cues and signals, you must be present for your baby. How you listen with your ears and heart, see with your eyes, and feel with your touch will affect the connection you are building through your caring touch.

Sometimes your baby will be telling you so much that it will sound like a story, a story that only she can tell. I am reminded again of Michael and Maria. Michael, just two months old, was so content when Maria massaged the heel of his right foot. He allowed her to stroke it, to move along the bottom of his foot, and make circles around his ankles. When she got to his left foot, however, she saw Michael differently than before. This time, as she began massaging his left foot, he began pulling it away, started to wiggle and fuss, and move his foot all about. He began protesting vocally, by making sounds that were not pleasant coos or babbles. He was telling mom something that at first she didn't recognize.

When I questioned Maria about Michael's hospital stay and any procedures performed on him, Maria was reminded that Michael was jaundiced at birth and that he went through many heel pricks to sample his blood, to make sure he was ready to be discharged home. Maria didn't know that the heel pricks had left any memory with Michael. From this experience, Maria learned that muscles have memory and that every baby's journey, from the beginning of their lifespan, leaves memories—pleasurable, non-pleasurable, or a combination of both. Unless those non-pleasurable memories are processed, they may stay with your baby forever.

Michael may be letting his mom know—as she stroked his left heel and saw him wiggle his foot, trying to move it away from her—that he remembered when he was in the hospital and received aversive touch. By reading this cue and following Michael's lead, Maria placed her hand on her baby, without using any massage strokes, but rather making that touch connection, listening and supporting her baby with her sympathetic ears, heart, eyes, and touch. By allowing Michael the opportunity to "vent," Maria was building bridges of love, respect, and empathy, which will carry them both on a lifelong journey, enhancing the parent-child connection that starts during infancy.

MAKING THE MOST OF YOUR MASSAGE MOMENTS

Positioning yourself for massage with your baby can occur while on a bed, on the floor with pillows and blankets, with your baby on a changing table, while you're holding your baby in your lap, holding your baby across your knees, or holding your baby in your arms as she looks out over the top of your shoulder. Massage may occur between you and your baby just about anywhere, in your home, in the car, on a plane, in the park, at a day care center, just as long as you and your baby are comfortable and willing.

You can decide what massage conditions meet your needs and the needs of your baby. After watching, waiting, and listening for a favorable response to the question "Do you want a massage?" you may reach for the massage oil. From previous experiences, you may have discovered such a good time for baby massage that you keep a bottle of baby massage oil near the changing table just in case a massage moment arises, or you may prepare to put together a little massage kit to hold all of the products that you need for massage. Just remember that babies become cold more quickly than adults, so check your baby's comfort level.

If you find yourself massaging your baby in a room, are you able to either raise the room temperature to ensure your baby's comfort, or can you cover the part of the body you are not massaging? Some parents like massaging their baby when she is wearing just a diaper, while others prefer when their baby is nude. If you remove all clothing, remember that it would be best to cover your infant's genital area with a loose diaper. Massage is so relaxing that your baby may easily urinate, and you may discover the true meaning of a flash flood as you find yourself wet and uncomfortable.

Where to Massage

There are so many places in which you can offer baby massage, but you must think outside the box. Massage, as mentioned previously, doesn't always happen in the home. You may be strolling in a park on a lovely day with blue skies, warm temperature, birds singing, and think, "Wouldn't this be the perfect time and place for my baby's massage?" Parents have told me that they have massaged their babies in a car, in a plane, on a boat, in a bath, on the changing table, on a mat, on the beach, on a hammock, and on a blanket, and in the company of a parent, a grandparent, an older brother or sister, a relative, or even a day care provider. If you are going to massage your baby in a room, then it is good to know about how to get the room ready.

Getting The Room Ready

If you choose to massage your baby in a room in your home, then here are ten simple steps to get ready. Make sure that you:

✔ Warm up the room so your baby will not be cold when she is undressed. Remember, baby's body heat escapes faster than an adult's does.

✔ Keep the room free from distractions—put your dog or cat out, and don't answer a ringing telephone.

✔ Have a CD player and CDs handy for added music, if not contra-indicated.

✔ Keep an extra diaper ready with handi-wipes and a change of clothes on hand for any urination. (Remember, massage relaxes babies, which can result in emptying the bladder.)

✔ Have liquid nourishment readily available, should your baby begin crying for it.

✔ Have an easily graspable toy (if your child needs to play with one during the massage time) or a pacifier readily available if your child needs to have one to suck on during part of the massage.

✔ Have natural edible oil in an easy-to-open bottle readily available prior to starting your baby's massage, so the oil will be ready when you are!

✔ Have some pillows available to put under your baby's head, or a soft blanket, comforter, or towel on which to lay your baby for creating a nesting area or swaddling.

✔ Take off any jewelry that may scratch your baby and wash your hands; keep nails on the short side so you don't poke your baby.

✔ Remove any harsh perfumes and let your baby smell your own body fragrances.

Getting Yourself Ready

For now, I will give you a sampling of suggestions for getting yourself ready to give your baby a massage. However, more will be explained in detail in Chapter 3.

To attune with your baby and acknowledge your baby, you must do the following to get yourself ready for massage.

✔ Relax yourself.

✔ Breathe deeply and allow your energy level to fill you in the presence of your baby.

✔ Ask your baby's permission to begin the massage using an upward inflection to your voice, or in a "parentese" question ask, "Do you want a massage?"

✔ Wait, watch, and listen for the response.

If Your Baby Signals YES:
Attune
Welcome Wonderment
Engage/Provide Massage
Read Your Baby's Cues
Follow Your Baby's Lead
Enjoy the Experience

If Your Baby Signals NO:
Make your baby and yourself comfortable.
Reposition your baby and yourself.
Check your baby's basic needs
  (diaper, nourishment, tired, sick, etc.).
Offer your baby a hug, cuddle, or toy.
Accommodate to meet your baby's needs.
Reposition your baby and yourself.

If Your Baby Continues to Signal NO:
Do not force baby massage.
Choose another time when your baby
  will be more willing.

If Your Baby Now Signals YES, then:
Attune
Welcome Wonderment
Engage/Provide Massage
Read Your Baby's Cues
Follow Your Baby's Lead
Enjoy the Experience

Preparing for Massage

We can maximize our potential when we are flowing freely and are in balance with our body's energy. What stretches or exercises does it take for you to relax enough so you may engage your baby with a massage? Will rotating your neck, or raising your shoulders up to your ears and then releasing them, give you enough movement to release tension from your body?

You may have a favorite exercise that you like that unwinds you. One of my favorite exercises is where I stand with my feet planted firmly on the ground with my knees slightly bent. Like a tree, I sense my roots going down from my feet deep into the earth, and I rotate at my hips a little. Or, I stretch my arms out as wide as I can with my palms facing upwards to the sky and I slowly rotate my head in a circular motion. Then I reach for the sky with one hand grasping the other wrist as I stretch out and lean over to one side, and then change hands and lean over to the other side, breathing deeply. You may find these stretches helpful, or you may practice others that work better for you.

Using various relaxation techniques, breathing deeply, and unwinding any tightened shoulder, neck, or back muscles helps you learn the importance of preparing yourself to connect with your child. Through touch, the first language of communication, you also learn that the massage experience can be pleasurable for you and your baby, and your bodies will look forward to the massage time together. Using breath as the energy upon which your body's energy rises and falls, you may watch your baby's breath and follow along with easy breathing to attune you and your baby in rhythmic harmony.

As you take the time to slow down your breathing and "become one" with your infant, you will notice how enjoyable the rhythm you've created can be. You will harmonize each time you and your baby rise in taking a breath. The two of you will be together in the moment. That is what massage is all about—and so is parenting: being able to lead and follow and adapt to your baby.

ARE ABBREVIATED MASSAGES OKAY?

Concerned parents ask me all the time if a shortened or abbreviated massage regime will work, especially when they don't have a lot of time to engage their baby in a full body massage. I remember Claudia, who wondered if she was going to be effective in giving a massage to her daughter Lily, when she didn't have enough time to offer her a full leg, foot, torso, arm, hand, chest, stomach, back, and face massage. Claudia didn't want "to do the wrong thing." But as you know by now, massage *is not doing to* someone; it is *being with* someone. So Claudia realized that being attuned interactively with Lily and showing Lily that she cared—even when there was no time for a full massage—by stroking, touching, and massaging fewer body parts would still make inroads into Lily's neuron highway. Claudia reported how alert and happy Lily was, every day, with just the simplest of strokes, such as rubbing her arms and legs while on the changing table.

Joe told me that he was so happy to have learned massage, and especially the strokes for a back massage, because whenever he came home from work he would first get permission from his son Damian for a massage, and then he would use the gliding stroke movement on his son's back. From only massaging Damian's back, Joe would feel Damian's entire body relax. Joe felt more competent as a parent by knowing a way to relax his son.

Similarly, Ellen reported that she gained a sense of confidence in

Harmonizing Your Movements

Did you ever marvel at the way a conductor leads the orchestra with rhythmic arm and hand movements, or how a violinist moves his arms through space holding a note for the exact amount of time that the songwriter had intended? Using your hands as a violinist uses his bow, you may begin to see a pattern of your own movement, the very same pattern that your baby feels receiving your touch. Do you prefer to use long or short strokes? Can you feel the firmness and gentleness of each movement? What is the quality of your movement? How light or heavy is it? Are you more apt to use a direct or indirect stroke? How fast do you massage your baby? What is the speed of each stroke; the quickness or slowness of each movement that seems most comfortable for your baby? With all of these questions, are you still able to follow your baby's lead and harmonize your movements with your baby's needs?

Sometimes you might think that your baby is so small that you must use a very light and soft touch. This may feel like a tickle to your baby. Vimala McClure, a pioneer in infant massage in the United States, encourages a stroke that is firm and gentle. Sometimes, with young babies, you may just hold your baby's leg or arm and not stroke them at all. This is called a "containment" hold. You are containing their body part without using any stroking. If your baby becomes agitated and upset when massage is provided, using this containment hold for several days or weeks may be most appropriate. Observe your baby's cues to determine when she is ready to move onto other stroke movements, gradually introducing them little by little.

knowing that when her twin boys were fussy in the hour-and-a-half-long car ride from the semi-rural area in which she lived to the Los Angeles basin, she could take off their shoes and socks and massage their feet. Using this abbreviated massage in the car, her twins would become calm and enjoy the rest of the ride.

There are so many wonderful stories from parents who have had great success by offering their child a brief massage when they didn't have time for a full body massage. They have said that even when they used the abbreviated massage techniques, by remembering to be present with their baby, feeling their breath attune with their baby's, and acknowledging their baby's needs, they felt connected with their infant and sensed their infant's enjoyment, too.

Some examples of places for abbreviated massages, as reported by parents, are in the car, in the bathtub, while lying on a bed, over the parent's shoulder, on a changing table, and while the parent is standing up. No matter how long a massage you are able to share, as a parent, not only do you reap the rewards while you are massaging your babies, you can

A massage need not be long to be effective.

reap other benefits as your children get older. (This will be further explained in Chapter 5.)

WHEN TO MASSAGE

Massage is individualistic to your lifestyle and your child's. Some of you are eager to massage your baby in the morning, and your baby is quietly alert right after waking up, making that a good time for massage. Others might have too much to do to get the other children off to school, or to get ready to go to work. For busy morning people, the evening time might be better.

Looking at the evening schedule, you may have more time available to offer your baby a massage after your baby's bath, and before sleep. Some parents use massage strokes during bath time, by rubbing baby's skin but making sure not to over-stimulate.

Sirah had several stories to tell about massaging her son Chance. She said how she usually massaged Chance in the evening after his bath. One afternoon, however, she offered him a massage to which he was quite agreeable. After the massage he slept for eleven straight hours. "This was the longest amount of time he had ever slept without waking," Sirah smiled.

Heather also told me how great massage was for Molly and herself after Molly's bath and before bedtime. Heather discovered it wasn't just her daughter who benefited from massage. She noted that, after the massage, not only was Molly more relaxed and able to sleep more deeply, but Heather reported her own breathing became deeper and she became de-stressed. She also had more energy to complete tasks at night and was able to stay up longer.

At first Steven enjoyed being massaged after his bath. As he got older, he enjoyed his massage in his bath. Together, he and mom Etty enjoyed many moments of pure joy and pleasure. Both mother and son benefited as Steven enjoyed his new routine, which led to a deeper and more relaxed sleep, which allowed Etty to sleep longer too!

As a parent, you can discover the time when your baby seems to enjoy her massage better than other times, and provide the massage during that time of day. But you need to note that just as your baby may go through a variety of different states, so too may she enjoy being massaged at different times of the day or night as she grows through infancy.

Rhythms change and cycles change, and parents must be keen observers of these differences, ready to be flexible with any massage schedule. The

For a massage, the optimum state for your baby to be in is the state of quiet alertness. In this state your baby is open to receiving you and engaging with you as she smiles with her eyes open and alert. She is not moving too actively or squirming.

most important thing is building the ritual of massage into your daily everyday routines and finding this special time to bond with your baby. You'll be creating memories, releasing endorphins, and spending pleasurable time with one another, which improves physical, cognitive, and social-emotional well-being.

CAUTIONS AND CONTRAINDICATIONS

It is always wise to check with your baby's primary healthcare practitioner to make sure that it is acceptable to offer massage to your baby. There are several medical conditions that are contradictory to massage, and you should refrain from massaging your baby when they apply.

DO NOT OFFER A MASSAGE WHEN YOUR BABY:

- Has a high fever

- Has an acute infection

- Has a skin disorder from either a contagious disease or inflammation

- Has had recent immunizations—wait forty-eight to seventy-two hours and don't massage on the area where your child was inoculated

- Has any abdominal difficulty

- Has any life-threatening medical condition

- Has the knot of the umbilical cord on—wait approximately two to three weeks for the end of the umbilical cord to fall off before beginning massage, as the umbilical cord area needs to be kept dry

- Has swollen lymph nodes

- Has a blood condition, such as blood clots

- Has any other acute illnesses or diseases

Not every contraindication is noted above, so the motto I tell parents when they ask me about a specific condition and whether to massage or not is, "When in doubt, check it out!" It is better to have a medical practitioner give the okay when you are in doubt, as this can prevent toxins from being sent throughout your baby's body, causing more disease or agitating an existing condition. Also, since you generally lie your baby down for a massage, it is best to follow these simple rules about massage and digestion: wait approximately one hour after a bottle is taken, and wait approximately half an hour after your baby is breastfed. In other words, wait for digestion to occur before giving a massage.

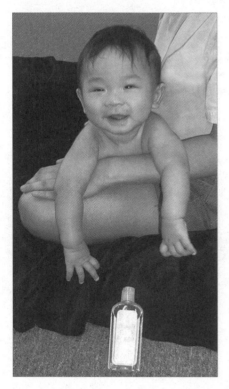

Look who is all smiles and radiant after receiving a smooth, silky massage with his natural baby massage oil.

USING BABY MASSAGE OIL

Using massage oil has more positive effects on newborns than not using oil. Infants showed fewer stress behaviors (clenched fists, grimacing) and lowered levels of cortisol (a stress hormone) following massage with oil versus without oil. It is better to use oil during massage, creating a frictionless touch between you and your baby.

A baby's uppermost layer of skin is still developing, and so it can absorb more than the skin of adults. Whenever you introduce a new product to your baby's skin, it is always important to do a skin test on your baby, to ensure that the oil you want to use will not be harmful. You can make up your own test by applying a small amount of the oil to your baby at least thirty minutes before the massage. Observe your baby's skin to note if any red blotches develop. If there is an allergic reaction, the blotches should go away in about sixty to ninety minutes. Baby oil that is natural, silky, light, and easily absorbed into your baby's skin is the best oil to use. In order to make sure that the oil used is the finest, these two quick lists can help you choose the best oil for your infant and you.

Oil Ingredients That Are Beneficial

❑ Natural ingredients

❑ Anti-bacterial

❑ Anti-allergic

❑ Non-scented

❑ Readily absorbed

❑ Edible oils (grape seed, sweet almond, sesame), but always administer a skin test prior to massage to rule out allergies

❑ Vitamin E

Oil Ingredients That Are Not Beneficial

❑ Mineral oil

❑ Scented oil

❑ Non-edible oils

Mineral oil does not readily absorb into the skin. Scented oils may camouflage the natural scents of the parents and caregivers, and non-edible oils may be harmful if ingested.

Should I Add Aroma to Baby Massage Oil?

Wherever you go these days, you are bombarded with smells! Perfumes are plugged into an electrical outlet to make your home smell like cucumber melon, or industrial scents cover up foul-smelling odors in an office building. You can smell harsh scents, fragrant scents, just about any kind of scent. You can go to just about any type of store and find scented candles, air diffusers, and sprays. No matter where we go, people are using fragrances to enhance their own smells or cover up bad odors. So why not use aromas with babies when you provide baby massage?

Your baby's skin is extremely sensitive, having more sensory receptors than that of adults. Babies are learning about their environment and about the people in it through their skin, which we know allows them to bond and feel secure with their environment. Studies show us that a five-day-old newborn, when given different breast pads from different mothers, can recognize the breast pad of her own mother by the smell of it! It is imperative for attachment and bonding that our own scent be identifiable.

There is no better way to start your life-sustaining relationship than with the incredible aromas of each other, allowing your baby the opportunity to know you and you, to know your baby. Baby massage oils are best when they are natural with limited aromas. So it is recommended that essential oils not be used with babies until they are approximately twelve months old, and still always check with your healthcare provider and an aromatherapist.

Your baby cannot tell you which aromas are or are not her favorites. It is, therefore, best left to Mother Nature to have natural scents and wait until your baby is approximately twelve months old to use massage oils with aromas or essential oils. Then, and only then, you will still need to make sure that you use the proper amount of essential oil in carrier oil, and use safety precautions with any ingredients that may require a skin patch test to insure no rash breakout.

BUILDING A LIFELONG FOUNDATION

Using the experiences provided by Kelly, Zuckerman, Sandoval, and Buehlman in *Promoting First Relationships* (2003), I have found that helping babies develop trust, security, and emotion regulation is just what baby massage easily parallels. This is done by providing love and attention every day; showing empathy and understanding; offering comfort when upset; providing a predictable world with rituals and routines; and providing play and exploration. Baby massage strokes are only one part of the whole. The entire way that you surround your baby with love; read her cues; allow her to lead while you follow; and speak, sing, or rhyme words during massage develops the loving, trustworthy, and secure relationship that leads to happiness, health, and relaxation.

Seven Simple Do's of Massaging Your Baby

1. Ask permission to massage. Respecting your baby is vital, so you want to ensure that you get permission to massage. Watching and listening to your baby's engagement cues allows you to be flexible and respond to your baby's state of being.

2. Follow your child's lead. If your child disengages and doesn't want a particular body part massaged, then move on to another body part that may be less stressful. Remember that some babies who have had hospitalizations and procedures to certain body parts (heels, stomach, etc.) may not be receptive to having that body part massaged. Do not force massage. Observe the behavior and introduce touch more slowly to that body part. Perhaps at first you can suspend your hands above the area so your baby can feel the warmth of your hands without putting pressure on the spot. Then you may be able to simply hold that body part or place your hand on the area without stroking it. Then your baby may allow you to use a brief stroke, and with repeated touches, fuller massage strokes may be tolerated and enjoyed by your baby.

3. Massage to relax or invigorate. Strokes away from the heart can be relaxing and those towards the heart, more invigorating.

4. Use your voice with words of endearment, encouragement, or questioning. Research shows us that baby massage includes other senses along with the tactile. By using upward-inflection questions or declarative statements using a "parentese" inflectional tone, or rhymes ("Do you want a massage?" or "You like when I massage your legs" or "Re-la-a-a-ax" or "This little piggy went to town . . ."), you are encouraging language development; auditory processing; vocabulary development; and strengthening both sides of the brain. (For more information, see Chapter 4.)

5. Eliminate distractions. Avoid distractions from television, telephone, pets, or other children that will interrupt the flow of the massage between you and your infant.

6. Massage the tummy in a clockwise position. This is so that you follow the natural excretion patterns of your child's "plumbing."

7. Massage for an appropriate amount of time. Brief massages with your baby may be all that your baby can tolerate, or all the time that you have, and that is fine. Sometimes a massage may just be several strokes on your baby's face to relax her, or on the shoulders to help integrate her with yourself.

As you build a lifelong foundation for your baby through baby massage, there are a few important points to keep in mind. As a quick point of reference, listed are seven simple do's and seven simple don'ts of massaging your baby that you might like to keep handy.

A baby's uppermost layer of skin is still developing, and so it can absorb more than the skin of adults.

Massage can occur over different time spans and in different places. The main tenet to remember is that massage is important for your baby and you. When reading your baby's cues and following your baby's lead, you provide respect and adapt your massage to your baby's needs. A massage

*Seven Simple **Don'ts** of Massaging Your Baby*

1. *Don't force massage onto your infant.* Sometimes infants who are crying may be doing so because of discomfort, such as gas bubbles, while other times your baby may be crying because she wants to stop the massage. If your baby has a gas bubble, you may need to massage her through the crying. If, however, the crying is a disengagement cue, then you want to give a massage break with a hug or a cuddle, a diaper change, or a feeding.

2. *Don't look for the perfect time to massage your baby.* You may not find it. You create the massage moments by your willingness and your desire, and your baby's willingness and desire.

3. *Don't use an oil that is too quickly absorbed into your baby's skin.* This may require more applications during the massage and interrupt the flow of the massage time with your baby.

4. *Don't expect your baby to immediately enjoy the massage.* Many times repetitive massages will be necessary before your baby associates the swishing of the oil in your hands with the relaxation and pleasure that is to follow.

5. *Don't worry if you don't know the exact strokes.* As long as you transfer your gentle and firm touch to your baby, she will receive the love and care you are sending, and feel secure and loved. Repetition will be your best teacher of strokes.

6. *Don't be rigid in your massage strokes.* Don't think that you have to follow a specific order of massage strokes. Your baby will be directing the body part that she wants massaged. One day she may enjoy her back massaged, and another day she may not. One day she may enjoy her face massaged first and another day, her legs. After you know the basic massage strokes, you will flow in your own massage movements and your baby will love them as your own massage signature.

7. *Don't feel that your child needs to be fully undressed.* Sometimes you may find yourself massaging through your baby's clothing as you massage her little tummy in a clockwise direction or stroke her back while you hold her on your shoulder. You may just be massaging her arms or fingers and find that undressing is not necessary.

of any length imprints experiences in the brain, which affect the releasing of hormones and endorphins; reducing of cortisol; utilizing of neuron pathways; and furthering of pleasurable memories. At the same time, it fosters the closeness and bonding that is so critical for your baby's growth, development, security, and trust. For many of you, baby massage may be new. Others may be seasoned professionals who want to learn new information about baby massage. I hope this chapter has given you more information and insight into getting ready for a massage, and all the steps that surround this preparation.

CHAPTER 3

BASIC STROKE
MOVEMENTS—
THE ABCs OF TOUCHTIME
BABY MASSAGE

Now that you have seen how easy it is to prepare for massaging your baby, get ready to learn about the simple ABCs while experiencing the AWE—Acknowledgment, Wonderment, and Enjoyment—of massage. Massaging your baby is a mutual experience, building confidence while strengthening your parenting skills. Dr. Elaine's TouchTime Baby Massage makes memorization of massage strokes easy by alphabetizing the names of the strokes for each section of the body. For example, when massaging your baby's chest, you would start with ABC—Attuning, Breathing, and Communicating—and continue with DEF—Dear Heart, Engaging Wings, and Fancy Circles. (The details of these strokes will be explained later in this chapter.)

There are many different massage strokes you can use when massaging your baby. I have chosen to use a variety of nurturing strokes that combine various movement qualities such as directionality, speed, rhythm, and pressure. Some strokes use long flowing movements while others use kneading movements; some strokes involve holding your baby's foot in your hand while others may have you holding your hands in suspension above your baby's body. Whether you start by massaging your baby's legs or by holding your baby's face in your loving hands, you will find out that the most important part of any stroke is not in the stroke, but in YOU! How you engage with your baby, read his cues, and nurture him through touch plays an enormous part in how your baby experiences his massage.

Humans are designed to be social. Since touch is the earliest communication link, massage fosters the earliest sense of sociability. During the massage you and your baby are linked in such a way that the union you enter into is bigger than the sum of your individual parts.

Imagine a captain of a sea vessel. Now realize that you will guide the massage like the captain steers his sailing ship. The captain adapts for changing weather conditions, while you adapt your movements to your baby's changeable moods. The captain learns the natural law of the power of the sea, while you will learn the natural law of the power of touch. Massage is not like learning to use a specific golf club for making a perfect par on a course rated by its degree of difficulty. There is no one specific nine iron or putter you can use in massage. Rather, these strokes are guides, with you making the decisions, as you follow your baby's lead of which stroke to use, when to use it, for how long, and with which rhythm, speed, or pressure.

Maybe your daughter will be like Eliyah, who at first didn't like her arms being massaged. Her responsive mom, Susan, decided not to aggravate her daughter by massaging her arms. Rather than gliding, she chose to hold Eliyah's hands in her own hands for a few minutes, gradually continuing to introduce more strokes while following Eliyah's lead. As you gain confidence using TouchTime stroke movements, you will find yourself moving beyond the strokes and beyond time, and, according to Leboyer, "touching the absolute with your very human hands." Let your hands be an expression of your endearment, without letting the nine iron or putter get in the way of your expression.

DR. ELAINE'S TOUCHTIME BABY MASSAGE—SIX SIMPLE STEPS

To help you recall the various massage strokes in this chapter, I've made it just like it was when you first went to school. You had to learn your ABCs and you probably experienced AWE with each new day. Every time you massage your baby, remember Dr. Elaine's:

ABCs

A	=	Attuning
B	=	Breathing
C	=	Communicating

in AWE

A	=	Acknowledgment
W	=	Wonderment
E	=	Enjoyment

A person's voice often changes when talking to a baby. This high-pitched, upward-inflecting voice pattern is known as "parentese."

A = ATTUNING

To attune is defined as to harmonize, be in tune, accord, synchronize, blend, sound together, prepare, and enable. Coming together with your baby through massage allows you to "fine tune" your relationship, promoting bonds and attachment, and furthering health and wellness.

When you attune, you are peaceful within yourself and close to your baby, allowing all the other distractions of the day or night to be put aside as you focus on one another. What a special time to begin your dance, your dialogue, with the magic of two people brought together through your primary sense—touch, the first language of communication.

Experience your baby's emotions. Sense your baby's feelings. Show your baby that you care. Let your baby know that you are here for him. Touch his little leg or tummy with a gentle firmness and use your "parentese" voice. Let your little one know how special he is and how much you love him.

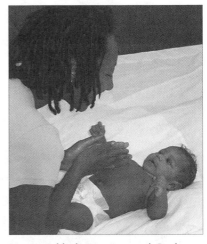

Mom and baby are attuned. Both exchange smiles and mom respectfully asks, "Do you want a massage?"

B = BREATHING

We take approximately 17,000 breaths a day. Dr. Andrew Weil, noted physician in mind/body medicine, tells us that "Eastern tradition views the breath as the vital link to prana, or the energy of the universe." Optimal use of the breath has shown to be beneficial for increasing circulation, lowering blood pressure, increasing energy, and reducing anxiety disorders.

During baby massage, energy is exchanged between partners paramount in establishing the rhythm of the parent-child relationship. Physically we breathe in oxygen and exhale carbon dioxide. We attune with our babies through the rhythm of our breath, our voice, and our touch. Breathing deeply allows our energy to flow, which helps to relax ourselves while furthering the connection being made between our baby receiving the massage and ourselves giving the massage.

I have put three letters together that form a word to help you remember the benefits of proper breathing. The three letters spell FAR. Proper breathing will enable your baby and yourself to go FAR, becoming Focused, Alert, and Relaxed.

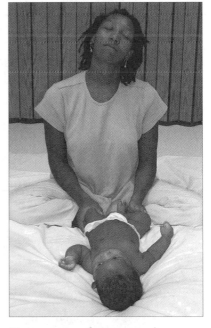

Mom prepares for massage by getting in touch with her own energy level, breathing deeply and savoring her time to unwind and relax while baby looks on.

C = COMMUNICATING

The sense of touch is our most social sense. When you touch another person, you are communicating. It is a sense that usually occurs with another person's involvement. When you are massaging your baby, your touch is worth a million words. (A picture is only worth a thousand!) The signals you are sending via your touch can be sensed by your baby. What you say and how you say it will be translated through your loving touch. This touch will translate into security and trustworthiness while providing a nurturing world in which your baby will thrive.

After asking your baby the question, "Are your ready for a massage?" you may rub your palms together with natural oil, allowing your baby to see your hands and hear the swishing of the oil near his ear. Your baby and you enter into this dynamic interchange. Memories will "kick in" and after several times of asking this question, your baby will begin to associate the sounds of your question and the sound of the oil swishing with the joy of touch, responding with a favorable "yes" to your question.

When you are massaging your baby, if you are like me, you will be in AWE—just knowing that you have either created this miracle before you (biological parent) or are witnessing a miracle (grandparents, adoptive parents, foster parents, and day care providers), and not forgetting that you are a miracle, too.

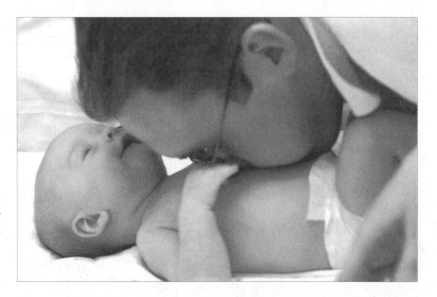

Dad's playful touch communicates his love and delight while his baby has so much fun giggling with daddy.

A = ACKNOWLEDGMENT

Acknowledgment is defined as recognition, acceptance, appreciation, giving thanks, and being grateful. The process of honoring another is vital in our daily life, as well as when you are massaging your baby. No matter how small, each baby is unique. No matter how big, each adult is unique. By asking, "Do you want a massage?" you are recognizing your baby as *someone* and not something, no matter how small. This reminds me of my square dance days, when before you would begin your dance, you would "Honor your partner" and "Honor your corner." So, too, in massage, we parent our baby from a place of respect, honoring the miracle he is and acknowledging the person he will become.

W = WONDERMENT

Wonder is defined as a miracle, amazement, a first-rate sensation; "Who would have thought it?" or "Will wonders never cease?" As you massage your baby, the dynamic interaction between you will bring you such wonder. See how massage calms your baby, relaxes your baby, facilitates your baby's sleep, rids your baby of gas, assists your baby's excretion, and builds a relationship while shaping your baby's brain and making you feel happy. Experience all of this while lowering your own blood pressure level and creating pleasurable memories. These benefits are truly miraculous—this is baby massage at its finest.

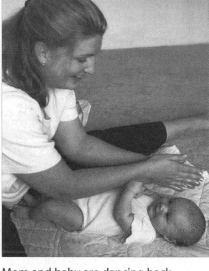

Mom and baby are dancing back and forth in their acknowledgment, wonderment, and enjoyment. Mom is swishing oil between her fingers, and baby is responding favorably. Let the massage begin!

E = ENJOYMENT

Enjoyment is defined as pleasure, euphoria, well-being, contentment, satisfaction, gratification, and "sweetness of life." No matter how much massage you offer, for whatever length of time, massaging your baby will release pleasurable hormones, reduce stress hormones in you and your baby's bodies and psyches, lower blood pressure, and enhance intellectual, physical, and emotional well-being. Oh, how sweet it is to find such pleasure in life, and to think you can have it on a daily basis with your baby!

STARTING OUT

Before you begin massaging your baby, remember that although you may be prepared and eager to start, your baby may be apprehensive at first, not knowing what to expect from your touch. Massage will be a new experience, and one that may take some time getting used to. Don't be disappointed if your baby doesn't seem too interested at first. With your continued encouragement and patience, while reading his cues, and gently reintroducing massage day after day, you will be delighted to find out how truly enjoyable massage becomes for everyone. Don't forget to check with your healthcare professional and make sure that your baby has no conditions that would prevent you from massaging him. (See Chapter 2 for more on contraindications.)

Your baby will "speak" to you with your back and forth dialogue. Your baby cares that you are with him, communicating and reading his cues. You know your baby best. As you massage your baby, you will come to learn which body part your baby most enjoys being massaged. You will also find out that if you begin with the same body part during each massage, your baby will begin to know that the massage is coming. This regularity will help prepare him for the rest of the massage, helping to establish everyday routines and rituals that assist in forming predictability, furthering security and trust.

Most parents I instruct follow the routine I provide of massaging baby's legs first (after the torso touch and energy rolls), which seems to be less obtrusive than massaging their baby's face. Other parents tell me that sometimes they will massage only one body part like the tummy to help relieve their baby from gas and reduce colic symptoms. You and your baby will be the judges of which parts of your baby's body to massage.

Kissing, cuddling, and holding your baby "speaks" to your baby just as your spoken words say "I love you."

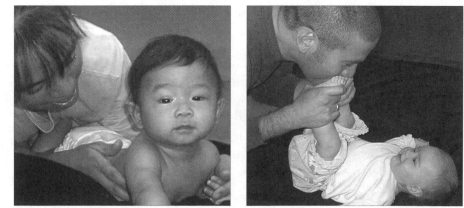

DR. ELAINE'S TOUCHTIME START TIPS

Many parents have told me when they first started massaging their baby they became discouraged and didn't know how they would ever fit another activity into their already busy day. Others told me that their baby was not too happy at first with particular massage strokes. Here are five Dr. Elaine's TouchTime START Tips to help your baby experience the joy of touch, and have your massage commitment remain resolute:

S = Stay encouraged. Don't let one bad day or experience get you down. Attune again and try again later that day or another day.

T = Take the time you have and use the time wisely. Don't expect to rush through massaging your baby without your baby noticing. If you are stressed, your baby will feel your stress and become stressed too. Tend to the here and now. Focus on being with your baby. Don't fret about the past or the future (the work you left on your desk or what you are going to make for dinner). If you are not in the moment, you can miss out on the valuable cues your baby is sending you and the enjoyment you are experiencing. An abbreviated massage is better than no massage at all.

A = Adjust and be flexible. Just because you massaged your baby in the morning one day doesn't mean that the next day you and your baby will be able to engage at the exact time again. Just because your baby enjoyed starting with his legs massaged on one day doesn't mean that the next day he will want to start at the legs again.

R = Recognize and follow your baby's cues. Your baby cannot "verbally" talk yet, but he has a large vocabulary without words. Watch your baby's body language and listen to the sounds he makes, so you can learn his readiness cues, his "time to stop" cues, and his time to "take a break" cues.

T = Talk to your baby as you massage him. Communicating through words facilitates your baby's listening skills; communicating through touch strengthens your parent/baby bond.

Taking Your Time

I am often asked, "How long does the baby massage take?" You and your baby determine the length of the massage. A full baby massage, depending upon the size of your baby, could take anywhere from fifteen minutes to half an hour. An abbreviated massage can take a shorter time, five or ten minutes. So if you only have limited time, it is best to concentrate on a few areas rather than rush through a full massage. Rushing will only bring forth anxiousness and impatience, translating into improper breathing and an unbalanced energy exchange, which can give rise to stress (releasing the stress hormone cortisol), rather than pleasurable feelings (releasing the "good feelings" hormones including serotonin).

Remember, just like everything in life requires flexibility, so does massaging your baby. I remember Katie, the mother of twins Sarah Jane and John. She said, "I started massaging Sarah Jane at twelve weeks of age. I was all ready to go and thought she would be too. It took her a few times to accept the massage and really enjoy it. I started out with only massaging her legs and after that very first massage she slept through the night! Now I can massage more of her body and she enjoys more and more each day."

Katie didn't say, "I have to massage every body part to see results." Rather, she massaged only her daughter's legs during the first massage and saw the immediate benefits—Sarah Jane slept through the night. Within days she moved onto massaging other body parts, such as Sarah Jane's arms and chest and then on to massaging Sarah Jane's entire body. On the other hand, Susan said, "Let's get real . . . I am glad if I can get in fifteen minutes of massage with my kids each day." When she does get in massage for those fifteen minutes, she is totally in tune with her babies and she enjoys the ritual it has become. You don't need to think that the massage time needs to be long to reap the benefits.

Another timing factor I am also asked about is, "What time of the day should I massage my baby?" Most parents tell me that they find the best time to massage their baby is after bath time when their baby is winding down from the day. They find that massage gives their baby the deeper relaxation he needs to get him off to a deeper and sounder sleep. Others have kept a journal to see the time of day that their infant gets "fussy" and massage their baby right before that time to help calm him or reduce his fussiness.

Timing also may change based upon your baby's stage of development. If you have an infant who is not yet sitting up, you will be able to lie your baby down on a soft mat or blanket and, with your baby's permission, offer a full baby massage. If your six to nine month old is sitting or rolling over, you may find that your baby may turn or roll over, changing the focus of your massage. And for your baby who may be starting to crawl, don't be surprised if he tries to crawl away from you. As your baby becomes more mobile, the amount of time that he will lay quietly on a blanket will lessen, and so your massage time may become shorter too. That "quiet alert state" that your baby will move into during early infancy may take a hike as your baby becomes more active, wanting to explore the world he lives in on his own.

Baby massage is a two-way street. No matter how much you want to massage your baby, never force a massage. There will be enough moments in your baby's life to offer massage when the timing is agreeable for both of you. Other times will present themselves as your baby becomes a toddler and moves into school and even adolescence. Just remember that you hold in your hands (and your heart, and your speech) the chance of laying a foundation of love and trust and respect through the art of massage at any stage of development.

YOUR PERSONAL TOUCH SIGNATURE

As a dance/movement therapist and former professional dancer, I find that when I am teaching parents or caregivers about massage and the various strokes they can use, I find myself also watching the type of movements they use with their babies. I see the quality of their movements, the way they shape their hands, the speed in which they move along their babies' bodies, the flow of their rhythm, the weight of their hands, the amount of space they use, their own breath, and their babies' responses.

Dr. Judith Kestenberg, Rudolph Laban, Warren Lamb, and Irmgard Bartenieff have written about the qualitative change in movement by patterns of effort (flow, weight, time, and space) and the form of movement—shape. Irmgard Bartenieff, choreographer (1970), and Judith Kestenberg, child psychologist (1965), expanded upon Laban's work. Their wisdom brings much to be thought about in relationship to baby massage.

As we shape our hands along our babies' bodies, we can watch our baby expand or shrink to our touch. We might notice the direction of the stroke movements, the amount of pressure on our baby's skin, and the speed with which we massage. The way we move along our baby's body will create a unique movement signature that no one else has. Our baby is journeying along our unique "rhythmical highway." Movements, breath flow, energy exchange, and intentional interaction (verbal and non-verbal) are all aspects of communication, and all aspects of Dr. Elaine's TouchTime Baby Massage.

Your baby senses your touch signature. Just like your own fingerprints, nobody else has your touch, your scent, or your voice. Your baby, even as young as three days old, can detect the unique scent of mother's breast milk when given a variety of soaked breast milk pads from which to choose. Dr. T. Berry Brazelton, noted physician and Professor Emeritus from Harvard Medical School, and Dr. Ed Tronick, noted child psychologist, showed how babies can also recognize both mother's and father's voices from the voices of others, moments after birth. In this same way, your infant recognizes the rhythmic patterns of your unique touch. It is your own touch signature that creates unique memories with your baby, memories that will span your lifetime.

MOVING AND SHAPING YOUR HANDS

You have an ability to form different shapes in space with your hands. Gravity allows your hands to move in different directions as you consciously, or unconsciously, use your weight for positioning your fingers, wrists, palms, and extending upward to your arms and into your shoulders, and back.

While your baby is a newborn or a few months old, you may find you massage your baby using one or two fingers of each hand. As your baby grows older you can add more fingers to your stroke movements, and eventually use your entire hand. The interrelationship among movement dynamics of effort, shape, and flow of your hands in space along your baby's soft skin, joined with your facial expression, tone of voice, chosen words, breath, and CARE (consistency, appreciation, responsiveness, and empathy), make up the extremely valuable elements of Dr. Elaine's TouchTime Baby Massage.

In the photos on the following pages, please remember that each time you see a baby being massaged, "it takes two." The emphasis is on the relationship between you and your child along with the use of movement. It's your touch signature in attunement with breath (energy), communication (spoken or unspoken words), eye gaze, voice inflection, turn taking, reading your baby's cues, following your baby's lead, and CARE that distinguishes Dr. Elaine's TouchTime Baby Massage from other massage techniques. Dr. Elaine's TouchTime Baby Massage is an avenue for attuning, bonding, developing and structuring the brain, and building secure attachments. Just as importantly, it is a cornerstone for creating a remarkable family of love, harmony, respect, and well-being.

You don't want to over-stimulate your baby, so watch your baby's cues. Baby massage is meant to be relaxing and enjoyable for both of you. There are many different types of strokes you can use with your baby. I have chosen to apply many of the the names of the "full efforts" that Rudolph Laban and his associates created. Following are the many different stroke movements you can enjoy using with your baby. The first two, Holding and Floating, are for when your baby is not able to tolerate your direct touch onto his skin.

HOLDING

Many times stroking a body part may be too over-stimulating for a newborn, a premature baby, or an infant. Having you support the weight of his arm or leg might be all that your baby can tolerate, until he can tolerate gliding. This may also be called a "containment hold."

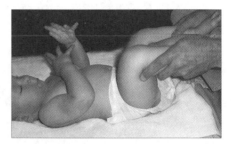

Holding

FLOATING

This stroke is indirect, light, and slow. Sometimes your baby will not be able to tolerate your direct touch on his skin. So you have an opportunity to hold your hands above your baby's body. The warmth of your own hands will permeate into your baby's skin as you hold your hands an inch or two above your baby's body. Sometimes at the end of the massage, if you end with his back, you might choose to finish with this type of stroke as you ease your hands off your baby's back.

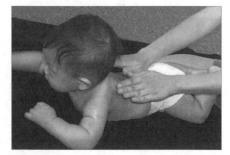

Floating

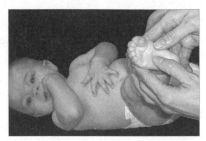

Pressing

PRESSING

This stroke is direct, strong, and slow. In this pressing motion, you can invite your baby's relaxation by using words that may instill calmness and ease (such as "so easy" and "relax"), or you may press the bottoms of your baby's feet or palms. Using the pads of your thumbs on the skin, gently and firmly apply pressure for a few seconds, hold it, then release, and move to the next point.

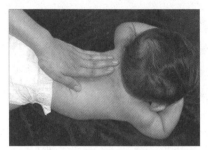

Gliding/Sweeping

GLIDING/SWEEPING

Throughout the massage you will find yourself using rhythmical stroking, sweeping, and flowing, linking each movement to the next. This stroke is direct and slow, but gentle and firm. Your palm may be used, or just your thumbs or index fingers when the space you want to massage is too small to accommodate your entire hand. This stroke is like effleurage, a long stroking motion that helps warm muscles.

SQUEEZING/KNEADING/TWISTING

Take both hands and curl your fingers around a leg or an arm and draw them together more snuggly. Then release the pressure and slide your hand down to the next area that is close to the spot that was just squeezed. This pressure feels like a "holding" and then a letting go. You may simultaneously squeeze and glide to make a kneading action like a kitten kneading its paws. If you are so inclined, you may add a little rotation to the squeeze and make a twisting motion, like wringing out a wet towel.

Squeezing/Kneading/Twisting

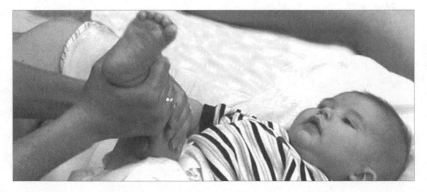

ROTATING/ROLLING

Your baby's fingers and toes love to be rotated or rolled. You can glide your finger down over each digit of your baby's toes or fingers and gently circle the finger or the toes, starting from the smallest digit and moving outward. This helps to separate the digits, and stimulates blood flow for your baby's reaching and grasping, and standing balance. Larger body parts may be rolled by placing your baby's leg or arm between your two hands and simultaneously rolling and gliding.

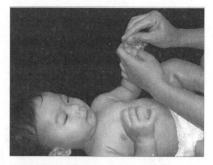
Rotating/Rolling

RUBBING

Using the pads of your fingers, you make small circular movements on the face, back, or buttocks. Rubbing is probably one of the most ancient types of massage strokes, dating back to China 3000 BC.

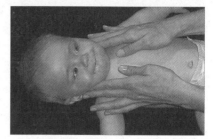
Rubbing

STRETCHING

This movement is done with a gentleness so as to be sensitive to your baby's range of motion and flexibility. You can use stretching in the yoga harmony exercises (explained later in this chapter), after your baby's muscles and tendons are warmed up from the massage. Be sensitive to the feel of your baby's joints, so that nothing is damaged.

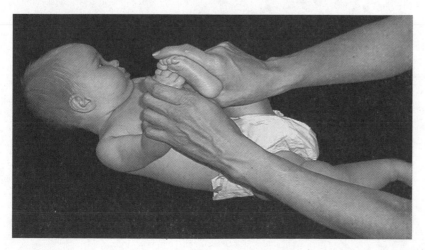
Stretching

QUICK AND BOUNCY STROKES

You will find out more about these strokes and massage for older children in Chapter 5. For now, when you are massaging your babies, your strokes are going to be slow, rhythmical, and sustained, rather than abrupt. When you massage your older child, you may use more percussive strokes. However, remember that the most important part of any massage is still YOU and your baby, the time you are sharing together, the relationship you are forming, and all the benefits of massage for the both of you. Other strokes that are quicker and more bouncy and brisk may be used with your toddlers and young children. Some of these strokes include dabbing, flicking, and even gentle "punching" (not too hard, of course).

Dabbing

This stroke is light, quick, and direct. It's a movement as if you were dabbing the perspiration with a handkerchief from your brow.

Move gently, quickly, and directly.

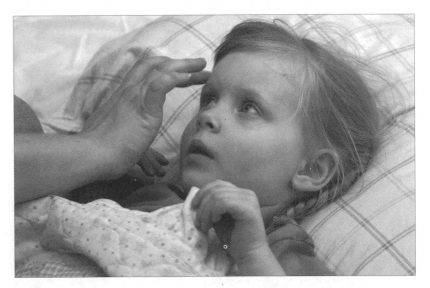

Flicking

This stroke is indirect, light, and quick. You use the sides of your relaxed hands and flick them away just as you touch the skin.

Gentle "Punching"

This stroke also uses relaxed hands, and lacks the intensity usually associated with "punching." Directly and quickly, gently bounce the top of your fist as you alternate hands. Pull your hand away as soon as it touches the skin.

LET THE MASSAGE BEGIN

In order for you to have an easier time remembering massage strokes when engaging in a full baby massage, I've created names that you can remember easily. Always begin massaging your baby with the ABCs (Attuning, Breathing, and Communicating) and just follow along with the remainder of the alphabet, D–E–F–G–H–I etc., until the strokes for each body part have been completed. For example, when you massage your baby's legs you would begin with A (Attune), B (Breathe), C (Communicate), D (Daybreak), E (Easy Squeeze), F (Friendly Five), G (Going Dancing), H (Happy Feet), I (I'm Moving Up), J (Jelly Roll and Joyful Touch), and K (Keeping It All Together). The alphabet strokes you would use when fully massaging your baby's back and neck are A (Attune), B (Breathe), C (Communicate), D (Divine Neck and Shoulder Rolls), E (Easy Glide), F (Fanning the Fire), G (Gentle Circles), H (Happy Wings), and I (I'm Moving Down).

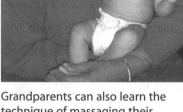

Grandparents can also learn the technique of massaging their grandchildren.

As you continually engage in massage, these strokes and names will become easier for you to remember. But this is not an IQ test. The relationship that you are forming with your baby through the massage is what counts. Your baby will feel your presence, experience your tenderness, and know you care. You are the most important person in your child's world. Enjoy your time together. You can always take an infant massage class if you would like more information from an instructor and to gain more confidence for yourself.

Begin Dr. Elaine's TouchTime Baby Massage by connecting with your baby using a Torso Touch. The steps are as follows, although I can't say enough times that massage is fluid; it is not rigid. These guidelines are never meant to be an end-all to the way you and your baby interact. Not every massage will be the same. Not every child will be the same. Remember all the pointers that have come before, and most of all, don't forget to have fun and enjoy this special time with your baby.

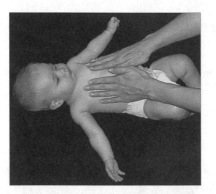

Attune with your baby with CARE. Using Torso Touch, watch your baby's state, breath, and mood, and connect through your touch.

Torso Touch (Warm-up)

- You have prepared the room or area for the massage.

- Your baby is in a quiet alert state.

- Your baby is lying on his back on a soft cushion, changing table, or bed, or is supported by nesting blankets wrapped together to form a little "nest" in which your baby is placed so he feels secure.

- Your baby is looking up at you.

- You begin attuning with your baby, watching his breath and his mood, and connecting through your touch.

- Take some easy breaths or rotate your head so you don't feel tight or stiff.

- Place your hands gently, with delicate firmness, on your baby's torso (center of his body), stroking directly and slowing down from the chest to his tummy.

- Use your "parentese" talk. You may say, "Daddy loves you," or "You are my boy," or any other phrases and words that are endearing.

- See if your baby is ready for a massage by asking, "Do you want a massage?"

- You will watch with your eyes, ears, heart, and touch, for the reply. When your baby shows you "yes" with his facial expression or body gestures, continue with the Energy Rolls.

Energy Rolls (Warm-up)

- Hold both of your baby's hands in the palms of your hands.

- Then, while smiling and talking to your baby, gently rub his palms with your thumbs. Do this a few times.

- You can include your "parentese" voice and add a short rhyme, such as:

    Fingers, fingers, oh so sweet,
    From your hands
    Down to your feet!

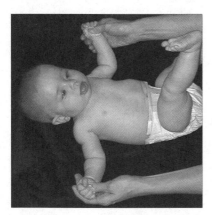

Baby senses mom's touch signature, hears her voice, and feels her heart as they prepare for their massage.

Remember you know your baby best! He may also like energy rolls on his feet or ears. Always remember to adapt your own strokes to your baby.

MASSAGING YOUR BABY'S LEG

Your baby's legs and feet are the foundation upon which he will eventually stand and walk. As your baby begins crawling, his feet and legs will propel him forward. It is important that he knows where his legs are in space, that he feels how his legs integrate with his hip joints. Massaging his legs assists in the development of leg tone, enhances movement, relaxes tense muscles, and brings body awareness to this body part. Your baby's legs integrate with the rest of his body, too. So, you may be massaging a physical body part, but what you are doing is going beyond the physical. I may speak about your baby's leg as the place of connection, but touching and massaging is more far reaching than just at the place of contact.

When massaging your baby's foot, you want to start with one foot and leg and when fully completed, move onto the other leg. You don't want to massage the upper thigh on one leg, go to the upper thigh on the other leg, and then move back to the first leg and massage the ankles, and then move to the other leg and massage the ankles. Always support your baby's leg and foot and keep them in alignment under his hip. Massage one leg completely before moving to the next leg. You want your baby to experience the full joy and integration of receiving a massage on one full body part at a time.

If you and your spouse (or significant other) would like to massage your baby together, you might choose to massage your baby's legs, and your mate might choose to massage both arms, rather than divide the legs and arms between the two of you. Each one of you has your own natural rhythm and movement signature. Be sensitive to the energy that you are imparting. You want to nurture your baby and be sensitive to his needs, rather than cause distress. Repeat each stroke about two to three times, unless a cue shows you that your baby desires more or less strokes.

Strokes for Massaging Your Baby's Leg

A = ATTUNING

- Be with your baby in the moment.

- Place your hands under your baby's buttocks, gently supporting your baby.

- Glide your baby's bottom parallel to the bed or mat he is lying on. (The action is like a glider, smooth and easy.)

- This movement helps to engage his full body from head to toe in preparation for the massage and moves the spinal fluid in the spinal column.

- Keep checking on your baby's quiet alert state.

It's like music when you attune with your baby, gently gliding the buttocks front and back. You also attune with your eyes, your voice, and your heartfelt touch.

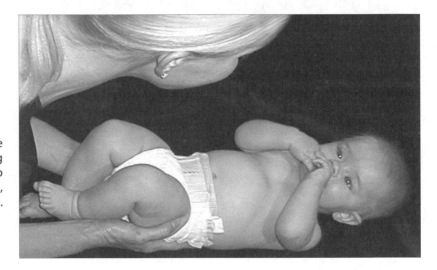

B = BREATHING

- Take a deep breath in and take a deep breath out.

- You could rotate your neck or do any exercise you find helpful to relax yourself, and have your hands relaxed, too, as you massage.

- Remember to breathe throughout the massage, harmonizing with your baby.

- Watch your baby's breath as you massage him, watching the expanding and shrinking of his ribcage.

Songs and Rhymes

Many songs and rhymes I have written for you to use appear in Chapter 4. Others appear later in this chapter. If the songs or music become too overly stimulating and cause disengagement, then, of course, refrain from using your voice, dim the lights lower, stop the music, and allow your baby an opportunity to regain composure and self-regulation. Take a cuddle break or a hug break. Start up again when your baby shows readiness, or end the massage and engage at another time.

"Gentle firmness" is a term that will be repeated often in the book. Massage strokes should be gentle, so as to not be digging into the skin. Strokes should also be firm—as opposed to being too light, which can cause a tickle on the skin.

C = COMMUNICATING

- Communicate through words and with your touch.

- Rub your palms together and swish the natural massage oil in your hands, placing them near your baby's ears so he can hear the sound and associate it with a massage.

- Or, have your baby see your hands swish in front of him as you ask permission. ("Do you want a massage?" "Can Mommy/Daddy/Grandma/etc. massage your ____?")

- Wait for an affirmative reply in gesture or word. Talk with your baby, recite nursery rhymes, and sing songs.

Daybreak is the time to wake up and enjoy the day, as you glide down your baby's leg from hip to toes.

D = DAYBREAK

- Use gentle firmness. Glide down from your baby's hip to his leg and ankle. Wrap your hand around his leg as you glide downward.

- Alternate hands, so you massage outside and inside your baby's leg.

- Watch your baby's cues and repeat massage with this stroke a few times.

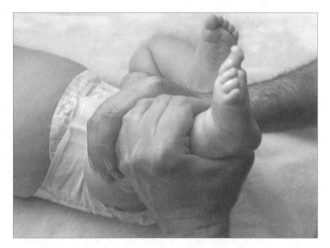

E = EASY SQUEEZE

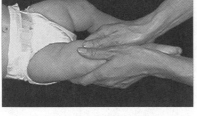

Easily knead your baby's leg from hip to ankle.

- Place both hands thumb to thumb, while using your fingers and hands to squeeze or knead down your baby's leg, starting from his hip.

- Then squeeze or knead again just below the spot where you began touching. Continue downward to the next spot that was not touched. Remember the age of your baby can affect the amount of touch he will tolerate. Strokes should be gentle, not digging into the skin, and strokes should be firm, not light enough to cause a tickle.

- Continue to knead or squeeze until you move down the entire leg.

- When you reach the foot, rhythmically squeeze all the way to the toes.

- Repeat this two to three times.

F = FRIENDLY FIVE

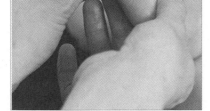

Rotate each toe and count to five to further your baby's cognitive skills.

- Place your baby's toe in between your thumb and index finger. Gently rotate each toe, stretch each toe out, and separate each toe from the other ones.

- Move from toe to toe.

- You can try the rhyme, "This little piggy went to market . . ." or you can make up your own rhyme or use mine:
  (Say each line with each toe.)

  > *Round and round we go*
  > *With your little toes*
  > *To the right and to the left*
  > *You are just the very best*
  > *B–A–B–Y!* (Hold the word "baby" as you add
  >   inflection and eye gaze.)

G = GOING DANCING

- Support your baby's foot in your hands.

- Press your thumbs, one at a time, moving up from the heel of your baby's foot to his toes, alternating your right and left thumb as you do this two-step. (There are thousands of nerve endings on the bottom of feet that travel to various internal organs. When you massage your baby's foot, his internal organs are also getting a massage.)

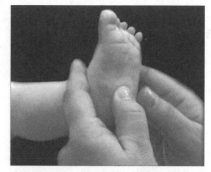

Pressing your thumbs up from your baby's heel to his toes will get your baby ready to "dance."

H = HAPPY FEET

- Hold your baby's foot with your two thumbs on the top, two index fingers lightly touching behind your baby's ankle, and middle fingers supporting his heel.

- Roll top of foot with the pads of your thumbs in little circles towards the leg.

- Continue moving outward, circling your thumbs around your baby's ankles.

- Continue holding your thumbs on the top part of your baby's foot as you take your index fingers and circle around the calf muscle and the bone in the heel.

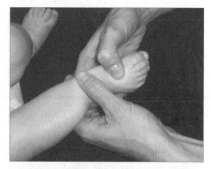

Roll top of foot with thumbs in circular motion toward the leg.

I = I'M MOVING UP

- Glide your hands upward from the ankle up the leg toward the hip. Your breathing and rhythmical movements allow your baby the experience of feeling safe and secure with your touch, as physically this upward stroke is sending the energy back towards his heart.

- Support your baby's leg with one hand (at the inside of the ankle). You are supporting your baby's leg as you hold it in the air, but not too high; just slightly off the ground so you can get under it.

- Gliding, stroke upward towards the hip.

- Fan your hand out around the hip with one continuous stroke.

- Alternate massaging the inner and outer parts of the leg with long, rhythmical movements.

- Repeat two to three times.

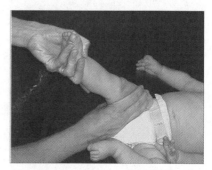

Glide from ankle up towards the hip, supporting your baby's leg and stimulating your baby.

J = JELLY ROLL AND JOYFUL TOUCH

Jelly Roll

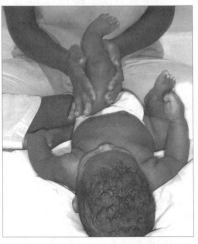

Roll your baby's leg between your hands starting at the ankle.

- Take your baby's leg between your two hands.

- Roll your baby's leg between your hands starting at the ankle.

- Roll up to your baby's hip.

Joyful Touch

- Press your fingertips on your baby's leg at the hip for about two to three seconds and then continue moving down towards the foot.

- In a soft, loving voice, you can say "enjoy" or "so calm" or "so easy" to relax your baby each time you move down the leg, several inches from the last press. (Moving down away from the heart is usually relaxing to your baby, while moving up towards his heart will usually be more stimulating.)

- Repeat two to three times.

K = KEEPING IT ALL TOGETHER

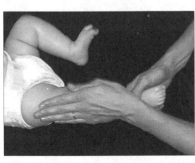

Press your fingertips at the hip for about two to three seconds and then continue moving down towards the foot.

- Sweep your hands from your baby's torso to your baby's legs in one gliding stroke.

- This stroke allows your baby to feel "whole" and connected, and signals a transition that you are going to massage another body part.

- Repeat one or two times.

Before massaging the next leg, remember your ABCs. Take some time between legs to breathe and relax as your energy and your baby's continue to attune, releasing pleasurable hormones, stimulating physical growth, and enriching emotional well-being. Before you massage the next leg, ask permission in a gentle voice ("Do you want a massage on your other leg?" or "May I massage your right/left leg?"). You may need to add some natural oil in your palm at this time. When you receive an affirmative response (smile, coo, alert look), proceed to massage the next leg with your natural oil.

The previous strokes are guidelines for you. You may find that there are too many strokes to use, if your baby is not ready for all of them yet. You can always skip some of the strokes. Just try to keep the balance so if you go down away from your baby's heart, try to end on a stroke that goes back up to his heart. Read your baby's engagement or disengagement cues (see Chapter 2), continuing or discontinuing the massage as directed by your ultimate teacher, your baby!

MASSAGING THE SIDES OF THE TORSO

Having had the experience of being a professional dancer also educated in dance/movement therapy, I am well aware that the human body is not flat! We are three-dimensional. That is why I like to massage the sides of my babies—not just their fronts or backs. I want "my babies" to experience the connection between their legs and their arms through the connection of their torso. Just like the Torso Touch was used to begin attuning with your baby before, I encourage you to use these torso strokes to bridge the space from your baby's legs up to your baby's arms.

Remember again your ABCs: Attuning, Breathing, and Communicating (see pages 66 to 67 for details).

D = DARLING BABY

- After the last "enjoy" or "calm" stroke (Joyful Touch), take both hands and move them up along the sides of your baby's torso.

- Glide upwards over the shoulders.

- Allow your fingertips to gently, but with firmness, stroke along the arm to the wrist.

- Give a little Energy Roll into the palms of the hand.

- Repeat two to three times.

- Follow your breath and watch your rhythm, flow, pressure, and speed.

- If you'd like, recite this little poem as you move up the torso:
    Darling Baby
    You're full of charm
    From your feet
    Up to your arms

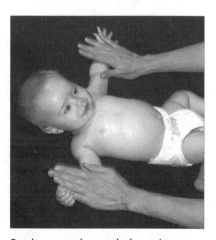

See how much your baby enjoys your gliding up from the torso along his arms to his wrists!

MASSAGING YOUR BABY'S ARMS

The arms are significant for our babies, as they explore their environments by reaching out into space, putting objects in their mouths, holding a bottle, or holding your hand. At the beginning of their lives, inside the womb, babies had their arms and hands covering their chests; therefore, at first when you go to massage your baby's arms and hands, he may be a little apprehensive, clenching his fists tighter than ever. As with all aspects of massage, approach each body part slowly, supporting each limb, giving your baby the opportunity to get used to your touch, and to warm up to the enjoyment he will feel after he is massaged.

If your baby is unsure of having his hands massaged, place your hands on your baby's arms and simply hold them there. You will begin to warm the skin, sensitize the skin, and continue to attune through the simple containment hold. As he becomes more comfortable, slowly introduce the strokes—perhaps one stroke a day, or sometimes one stroke a week. Never force your baby. Never demand that your baby be massaged. In time, your baby will enjoy you massaging the body parts he may have not initially enjoyed having had massaged.

Shannon noted how Stacey, at first, did not like her arms massaged, and pulled them away every time she tried to massage them. Shannon realized that by going more slowly and just placing her hand on her daughter's arm, Stacey became more comfortable having her arm touched and eventually permitted her mom to massage her arms, smiling all the time. Cole was another baby who, at first, resisted being touched, so his dad played a game with him. First he kissed his hand. Then he brought over a stuffed animal and rubbed Cole's hand on the soft Barney. Soon, Cole opened his hand to touch Barney, and this allowed dad to massage his hand. With subsequent games and strategies, Cole began allowing dad to massage more. Eventually, Cole allowed his hands and arms to be massaged, along with the rest of his body.

Strokes for Massaging Your Baby's Arms

For the most part, the strokes for your baby's arms will be the same as the strokes for his legs. Remember your ABCs in AWE.

D = DAYBREAK

- Use gentle firmness. Stroke down from your baby's shoulder to his arm and wrist.

- Wrapping your hand around your baby's arm, glide downward while supporting the wrist with the other hand.

- Alternate your hands so you massage outside and inside your baby's arm.

- Watch your baby's cues and massage two to three times, more or less.

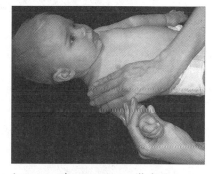

Wake up your baby's arm with gentle firmness from his shoulder down his arm to his wrist.

E = EASY SQUEEZE

- Place both hands thumb to thumb while using your fingers and hands to rhythmically squeeze your baby's arm, starting from his shoulder.

- Knead your fingers down to the next spot that was not touched.

- Continue as before until you squeeze down the entire arm.

- Repeat two to three times.

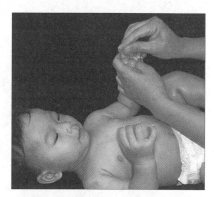

Just a tender squeeze will do it.

F = FRIENDLY FIVE

- Placing your baby's fingers in between your thumb and index finger, rotate each finger, stretch each finger out, and separate each from the other ones.

- Move from the small finger (pinky) to the thumb.

- You can try the rhyme; "This little piggy went to market . . ." or you can make up your own rhyme or use mine.

(Say each line with each finger.)

> *Round and round we go*
> *With your finger so*
> *To the right and to left*
> *You are just the very best*
> *B–A–B–Y!*

(Hold the word baby as you add inflection and eye gaze.)

Separating each finger will make it easier for your baby to grasp objects and eventually point.

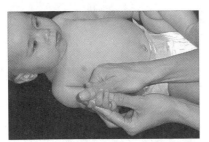

Alternate your thumbs as
if you are dancing right
inside your baby's palm.

G = GOING DANCING

- Support your baby's hand (holding at the elbow).

- Alternate your right and left thumb as you do the two-step,
  pressing from the base of your baby's palm, stepping up to the
  fingers.

- Repeat two to three times.

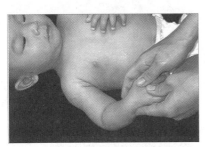

By rolling the top of your baby's
hand with your thumb pads in little
circles, your baby gains awareness.

H = HAPPY HANDS

- Support your baby's hand with your two thumbs on the top
  and two index fingers lightly touching your baby's palm.

- Roll the top of the hand with the pads of your thumbs in little
  circles, towards your baby's wrist. (Right thumb moves clockwise and left thumb moves counterclockwise.)

- Use your index fingers to circle around your baby's wrist. (Right
  thumb moves clockwise and left thumb moves counterclockwise.)

- Repeat two to three times.

I = I'M MOVING UP

This movement helps your baby
experience the connection between
his wrist, arm, shoulder, and back.

- Support your baby's arm with one hand (at the inside of the
  wrist).

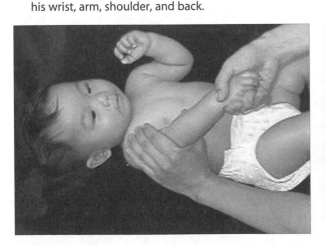

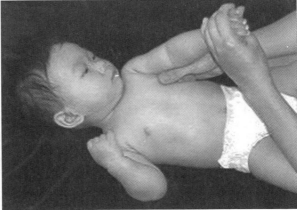

- Gliding, stroke towards the shoulder with the other hand. Your breathing and rhythmical movements continue to allow your baby the experience of feeling safe and secure with your touch, as physically this upward stroke is sending the energy back towards his heart.

- Fan out around the shoulder with one continuous stroke, feeling the back part of the shoulder.

- Alternate massaging the inner and outer parts of the arm with long, rhythmical movements.

- Repeat two to three times.

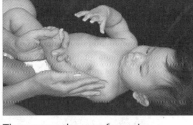

First roll arm between hands starting at wrist up to shoulder.

J = JELLY ROLL AND JOYFUL TOUCH

Jelly Roll

- Take your baby's arm between your two hands.
- Roll your baby's arm between your hands, starting at the wrist.
- Roll up to your baby's shoulder.
- Repeat two to three times.

Joyful Touch

- Press your fingertips on your baby's arm at the shoulder for about two to three seconds, and continue moving down towards the hand.

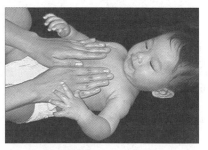

Then press the arm from the shoulder to the hand.

- In a soft, loving voice, you can say "enjoy" or "so calm" or "so easy" to relax your baby each time you move down the arm, starting from a spot a couple of inches from the last press.

- Repeat two to three times.

K = KEEPING IT ALL TOGETHER

- Sweep your hands from your baby's torso to your baby's legs in one gliding stroke, providing a unity touch.

- This stroke allows your baby to feel "whole" and connected, integrating your baby's body image and signals a transition that you are going to massage another body part.

- Repeat one to two times.

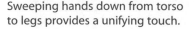

Sweeping hands down from torso to legs provides a unifying touch.

MASSAGING YOUR BABY'S CHEST

The chest houses many organs and glands: the lungs, vital for breathing and vocalizing; thymus and lymph glands, for health and immunity; and the heart, our body's largest pumping machine and holder of emotions. The heart is an energy center (chakra) linked in Eastern tradition to balance, harmony, and coping with loss. Many times while you are massaging this body part, your baby may begin vocalizing as if telling you a "story." Listen attentively, allowing your baby the opportunity to "get something off his chest." Respectfully listening to your baby helps you bond and furthers your relationship.

Strokes for Massaging Your Baby's Chest

Remember your **ABCs** in **AWE.**

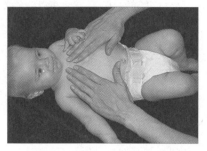

Let your fingers glide from your baby's chest diagonally across and off at your baby's torso.

D = DEAR HEART

- Place your fingertips on your baby's chest, pointing in a diagonal with your index fingertips touching and your thumbs end to end so as to form an upside down heart. Your thumbs should meet above your baby's navel so that you are focusing this stroke on your baby's chest. Your other fingers are pointed towards one another.

- Let your hands glide from your baby's chest at the arm level, diagonally across the chest and the sides of your baby's torso.

- When your hands get down to about your baby's waist, let them come up off the body.

- Repeat two to three times, more or less depending upon your baby's cues.

- With each glide across your baby's chest, lovingly say "my dear heart."

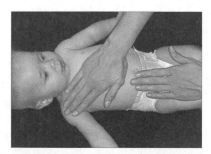

Gliding rhythmically and diagonally, criss-cross your baby's chest from the hip to the opposite shoulder.

E = ENGAGING WINGS

- Gaze into your baby's eyes.

- Glide your right hand from your baby's right hip diagonally up across your baby's chest to the opposite shoulder, and massage that shoulder gently.

- Repeat with your opposite hand gliding rhythmically, criss-crossing your baby's chest.

- This is the time that your baby may "tell his story." Be prepared to listen. You may say, "tell me more," or "tell me what you think."

- Repeat two to three times.

F = FANCY CIRCLES

- Place both hands, gently and with firmness, on your baby's chest with thumbs and index fingers touching. (Depending on the size of your baby, you may use one finger, two fingers, or your whole hand.)

- Simultaneously glide or rub your right and left hands in a circular motion on your baby's chest, around each nipple with your right hand "waxing on" (moving clockwise) and your left hand "waxing off" (moving counterclockwise).

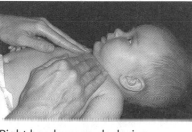

Right hand moves clockwise and left hand moves counter-clockwise around the nipples.

- Follow the rhythm of your breathing.

- Here is a poem you can recite while you are drawing your fancy circles:

> *Fancy circles on your chest*
> *Going east and going west*
> *You're the one I love the best*
> *Fancy circles on your chest!*

G = GENTLE BREEZES

- Finish the chest by using gentle relaxation strokes, sweeping both hands down the sides of your baby's trunk.

- Glide from the shoulders to the toes, gliding your hands downward in synchrony, gently following the contours of your baby's trunk, hips, and legs.

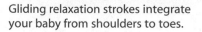

Gliding relaxation strokes integrate your baby from shoulders to toes.

- This unity stroke unifies your baby by bringing all of the body parts together, preparing your baby for the next transition.

- Repeat two to three times.

MASSAGING YOUR BABY'S TUMMY

Next to your baby's chest, your baby's stomach and intestines are delicate structures. Like other bodily systems, your baby's stomach and intestines continue developing outside the womb. That is why so many newborns and young babies have difficulties with digestion and elimination. Their "plumbing" is not fully developed and just as you expect your own household plumbing not to back up, so too, you expect your baby's intestines to be functioning smoothly to rid his body of any waste products. Sometimes reality doesn't meet our expectations.

Some babies are unable to digest their caloric intake, building up gas and causing stomach pain. Many parents are not aware of just how much gas their baby is holding inside. "John doesn't really have any gas," said Gary, as he began massaging John's tummy. Gary was the first one to get a whiff of the odor his baby released. Surprise, surprise—he didn't have a handkerchief to cover his nose. So many parents don't have the foggiest notion that their baby is retaining gas, causing discomfort and pain, and that massage will make their baby feel so much better when the gas is released. Gary discovered that it wasn't that his son didn't have any gas; it was instead a question of, "How much?"

Other babies may become constipated. (I will discuss special strokes to ease the conditions of colic, gas, and constipation in Chapter 6.) The tummy houses your baby's "inner plumbing" with its natural flow via gravity. Go to different countries and you will find the drain empties in a clockwise position above the equator and a counterclockwise position below the equator. To prevent your baby's plumbing from backing up, always remember to massage your baby's tummy like the hands of a clock going clockwise.

Give your baby a chance to digest his milk before you massage him; wait approximately thirty minutes after having breast milk and wait at least forty-five minutes after taking in formula. Adjust these times according to your own infant's needs.

Strokes for Massaging Your Baby's Tummy

Remember to follow the **ABCs** in **AWE** for massaging your baby's tummy.

D = DADDY LONGLEGS

- Start at the level of the belly button from the 9:00 to 3:00 position of an imaginary clock on your baby's tummy. Imagine the handles are at the level of the belly button.

- Walk across your baby's tummy compassionately and firmly; alternate pressing and releasing the flat part of your index finger with your middle finger, rhythmically moving any bubbles out. Make sure that you keep continuous pressure so that no gas bubbles get away.

- Repeat three to four times.

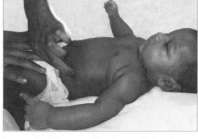

Let your "fingers do the walking" as you get any gas bubbles out!

E = EARTH WATCH

- Place the flat of your right hand at your baby's navel and tummy.

- Place the flat of your left hand next to your right hand.

- In a clockwise position, rub your hands firmly over your baby's tummy, circling round and round like the shape of our planet Earth, leading with your right hand and following with your left.

- Keep your hands on your baby's tummy; don't lift up.

- Repeat about three to four times.

- If you want to and your baby is agreeable, you can alternate the Daddy Longlegs stroke with the Earth Watch stroke, and repeat the series three to four times.

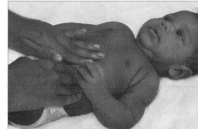

Circle your baby's tummy round and round, with your left hand following your right.

F = FUN GALORE—LEGS DOWN LOW

- Place one hand in the center of your baby's tummy below the rib cage, and pretend to be smoothing sand from the beach and building a sandcastle.

- Use the outer edge of your hand to "scrape the sand" and lower down the rest of your hand (beginning with your pinky, ring finger, middle finger, index finger, then thumb) flat onto your baby's tummy and release.

- One hand alternates with the other.

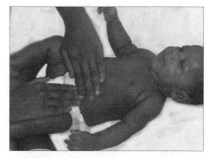

Smooth your baby's tummy by using the edge of your hand from the pinky to the index finger and alternating one hand with the other.

- Make sure that one hand always has contact with the stomach, for continuity and to keep the flow of energy moving.

- Watch your rhythm and your movement pattern, to ensure that it is not too fast or too slow.

- If your baby has difficulty with gas, he may not like this stroke at first, so you may want to start with a lighter touch and build into a deeper one. If your baby has lots of gas, you can use the stroke pattern described in Chapter 6.

- Repeat two to three times.

F = FUN GALORE—LEGS UP HIGH

- Support your baby's legs at the ankles with one hand and your middle finger separating the feet.

- Lift legs while the other hand "builds" sandcastles. This position allows you to go deeper into the tummy than the Fun Galore—Legs Down Low stroke movement alone, but make sure that your baby's hips stay on the floor and even when supporting the ankles.

- Repeat two to three times.

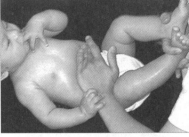

Keep baby's hips on the floor as you bring both legs up, allowing your hand to move more deeply into baby's tummy area.

G = GENTLE BREEZES

- Finish massaging your baby's tummy by using this gentle calming and harmony stroke, sweeping both hands down the sides of your baby's trunk.

- Glide your hands downward in synchrony, gently following the contours of your baby's tummy, hips, and legs.

- This unity stroke unifies your baby by bringing all of the body parts together, preparing your baby for the next transition.

- Repeat two to three times.

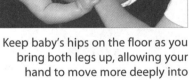

Calm your baby and bring harmony with this unity stroke gliding your hands down your baby's trunk, tummy, hips, and legs.

MASSAGING YOUR BABY'S BACK AND NECK

The back may hold lots of tension. Usually by the time your baby has his back massaged, he is ready to relax more deeply. So many parents tell me how they love massaging their baby's back because they know that he is going to sleep soundly. Also, since massaging your baby's back will require that you place your baby on his tummy, this will provide your baby will valuable "tummy time." Babies have been being put down to sleep on their backs since the SIDS epidemic. That means that unless you make a specific time to put your baby on his tummy, he may not have enough experience in that position, which is so needed for head and neck strengthening, and weight bearing. Also, this position may feel awkward and strange, and you may find your baby voicing protest about being on his tummy.

Using baby massage will help your baby become more comfortable in this tummy position. This position is considered a developmental necessity as it is from this position that scooting and crawling emerge. I remember Joe reported how much Nicole didn't like having her back massaged because she didn't like being on her tummy. After several attempts she relaxed more and engaged with her dad. She took off crawling soon thereafter. Joe was happy and glad that he hadn't given up on massaging his daughter's back. I'm sure Nicole was happy too!

Read Your Baby's Cues

One thing that distinguishes Dr. Elaine's TouchTime Baby Massage is that my techniques are flexible. You, the parent, know your child best. At this point in the massage routine, after massaging your baby's tummy, I invite you to determine the next strokes with your baby. By reading your baby's cues, and knowing how much time you have, you can determine which body part your baby would like to have massaged. If we are going to use the yoga harmony exercises, then massage baby's back, turn him over to end the massage with him facing up. Or, if your baby is ready for a change in position, you can turn your baby over and massage your baby's back.

Sometimes, however, your baby may look so relaxed that you may be able to continue massaging him lying on his back, and then change his position after you have massaged his face and head. Massaging his back after his face and head could then end in his drifting off to sleep. Since I value the rhythm and flow of massage, and the relationship building that is occurring, I will present the strokes for massaging your baby's back at this time. Just know, however, that you have the choice to reduce strokes, add strokes, or change strokes throughout the massage. As I have said time after time, these are guides. You know your baby best, and you are in charge of following your baby's lead.

Strokes for Massaging Your Baby's Back and Neck

Remember your **ABCs** in **AWE.**

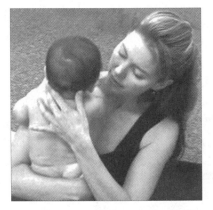

Mom divinely rubs her baby's neck in a circular motion with her left fingers while supporting him with her right hand.

D = DIVINE NECK AND SHOULDER ROLLS

- Hold your baby in your arm, or have your baby lying tummy down on a soft mat, or lying over your knees.

- Use the pads of your fingers. If your baby is in your arms then you will use one hand.

- Gently and firmly rub the pads of your fingertips in a circular motion on your baby's neck on either side of the spine.

- Repeat with small circles two to three times.

- Gently and with firmness use the pads of your fingertips in a circular motion on your baby's shoulders.

- Repeat with small circles two to three times.

E = EASY GLIDE

- Glide one hand from your baby's neck down to the buttocks and down to your baby's toes.

- Alternate your hands.

- Glide two to three times.

Glide one hand down from your baby's neck to his buttocks and then to his toes in one easy glide. This will feel so soothing.

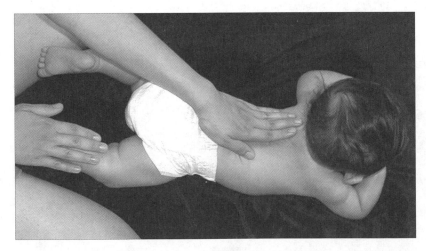

F = FANNING THE FIRE

- Take both hands and lay them gently on your baby's back.

- Slightly angle your hands outward.

- Glide the hands away from the center of the back as if smoothing out a velvet cloth.

- Bring hands back to the center of your baby's back.

- Allow your hands to rhythmically and gently move down your baby's back. Each time your fingers will go lower than they were before.

- Repeat two to three times.

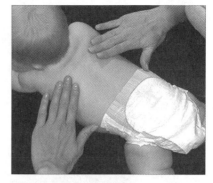

Glide your baby's back as you fan your hands from the center outwards.

G = GENTLE CIRCLES

- Take your index fingers (or two or three fingers depending on your baby's size and the size of your fingers), and simultaneously make little circles on the right and left of the spine, starting at the base of the neck. Finger(s) on your right hand will move clockwise. Finger(s) on your left hand will move counterclockwise.

- Circle next to the spine but not on the spine.

- Go down to the bottom of the spine, inching slowly down with both fingers at the same level of the spine.

- Keep circling into the buttocks.

- Repeat three or four times.

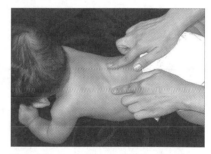

Simultaneously make little circles clockwise and counterclockwise on the sides of your baby's spine.

H = HEAVENLY WINGS

- Place one hand on the hip of your baby as he lies on his tummy and glide that hand diagonally up to the opposite shoulder, as if outlining a wing of an angel.

- Allow your hand to glide over the shoulder blade so it gently massages the front of the shoulder.

- Repeat with the opposite hand, from the opposite hip.

- Repeat two to three times.

- Watch your baby's back relax as you follow the rhythm of your breath.

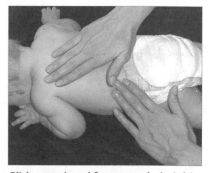

Glide your hand from your baby's hip diagonally to his opposite shoulder and over his shoulder blade.

▌ = I'M MOVING DOWN

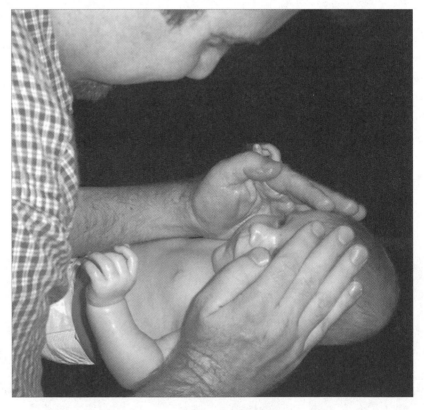

Relax your hands as you glide down your baby's back, getting lighter and lighter with each stroke.

- Allow your hands to be relaxed, with your fingers opened, gliding down along your baby's sides and back.

- Gently stroke and glide downward from your baby's neck, along his sides, and down to his feet.

- Repeat two to three times.

- Each stroke can get lighter and lighter with a finishing touch.

- Hands may be suspended above your baby's back (Floating). Each one of these last strokes will assist with relaxing your baby, eventually sending him off to sweet dreams and a peaceful sleep. Some parents like to use the back strokes before putting baby to sleep.

- Take a moment to breathe deeply, and sense the same type of calm your baby is experiencing with this finishing stroke.

Acknowledging your baby as a gift from the divine, hold your baby's head gently with your fingertips along the side of his face and the base of your hands along his jaw.

MASSAGING YOUR BABY'S
HEAD AND FACE

At the beginning, your baby may not want to have his head or face massaged. For many babies, this was the first part of the body that came into the world. By always reading your baby's cues, you will know whether he is or is not receptive to having his head or face massaged that day. The top of your baby's head will feel soft where the fontanels—the bones of your baby's skull—have not joined completely. This softness was needed to be able to get your baby's head through your birth canal. The back fontanel usually closes by about four months of age and the front fontanel usually closes between nine months and eighteen months of age. I do not recommend directly massaging on top of your baby's skull, until your baby is older and the spots have closed or the very tough protective membrane has had a chance to grow.

Always approach your baby's face with care, considering there are so many sensory points on the front and side of the face (eyes, nose, mouth, and ears). You may want to kiss your baby's face. You may need to hold your baby's face gently, and lovingly talk to him before he will give you permission. Again, let your baby instruct you on the best way to approach, and what parts of his face he likes being massaged. In due time, he will allow more and more face massage, if he doesn't at first.

For instance, Heather was born after a hard labor. Whenever Sheila would want to massage her face, she fussed and cried and would have nothing of it. Sheila listened empathetically to her daughter and understood the trying time they both had had during the delivery. So she started with the holding stroke, and just placed her hands on the side of Heather's face. At first Heather frowned and moved her head from side to side. Within several days, however, she got used to the sensation of her mother's hands on the side of her face, and she let Sheila stroke her forehead for the very first time.

Whether you are using several fingertips, or one fingertip at a time, when you massage your baby's face you *do not* need to use oil. Your baby doesn't need oil to be placed on his face, as it may get into his eyes, and your hands probably have enough oil remaining on both your hands and fingertips from massaging other body parts.

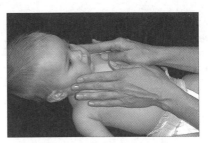

Relaxing the muscles of the man-dibular joint is a great way to reduce tension in your baby's muscles that are used for sucking and swallowing.

Strokes for Massaging Your Baby's Head and Face

Remember your **ABCs** in **AWE.**

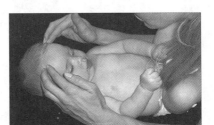

D = DIVINE PRAYER

- Hold your baby's head in a type of prayer pose as you place your fingers along the side of your baby's face and the base of your hands along his jaw.

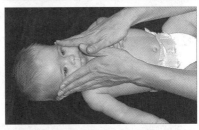

E = ELAINE'S HEARTS

- Put your fingertips at the center of your baby's brow in between the eyebrows, above your baby's nose.

- Gently move your fingertips (number will vary depending on the size of your baby's face and your hands) up to the place on your baby's forehead that is sometimes thought of as your "third eye."

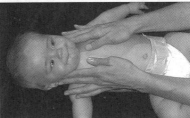

Envision making a heart on your baby's face starting at your baby's brow and gliding downward from his forehead, temples, and cheeks to the bottom of the jaw.

- From this position, move your hands over your baby's fore-head, down the temples, along the sides of his cheeks, and down to the bottom of his jaw.

- This stroke is as if you are making the shape of a heart on your baby's face.

- Repeat about two to three times.

- You can say a little rhyme with this movement too:

  Hi, Baby, I see you
  Such a pretty, pretty, face
  How do you do?
      Or
  Hi, Baby, I see you
  Such a happy, little, face
  I love you!

F = FUNNY FACES CHEEK CIRCLES

High

- Take one or two fingertips of each hand and rub in small circles on your baby's cheeks.

- See how big you can make the circles, or how small, and watch how your baby tolerates your touch.

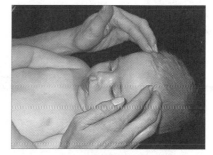

Gently rub outward along your baby's temples with your fingertips, which is so soothing for the face.

(One note of caution: for younger babies, one to three months of age, the rooting reflex is still strong. A rooting reflex is a newborn's natural reaction to your stroking of his cheek or the side of his mouth. Your infant turns his head to the side that was touched in his survival mode of rooting onto the something to suck. Be observant; if he begins to root you may want to stop the stroke.)

Low

- Continue to make circles with your fingertips on the mandibular joint (the hinge where the mouth opens). With your baby usually sucking so much, this is a great way to relax these muscles.

Tender Stretches

- Place one or two fingers on the middle of your baby's cheek and gently move apart to stretch the cheek.

- Repeat on other cheek.

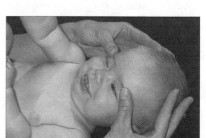

Gently dab your fingers along your baby's temples and let your fingers "do the walking."

Temple Touches

Temple Rubbings

- Place your fingertips on your baby's temples.

- Gently rub temples outward.

Temple Footprints

- Place your fingertips on your baby's temples.

- Gently dab your fingers on his temples.

- Repeat this two to three times.

Blocked sinuses can cause great discomfort when fluids don't drain and pressure builds up. Gently allow your fingertips to glide across your baby's brow, above the eyes and outward to the temples.

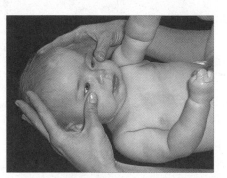

Blocked sinuses can occur below your baby's eyes, too, so be sure to sweep both high and low.

Sinus Sweep

High

- Gently place both sets of fingertips at the center of the forehead.

- Allow your fingertips to glide across your baby's brow, above his eyes outward to the temples.

Low

- Gently place both sets of fingertips under your baby's eyes.

- Allow your fingertips to glide under the eyes toward the ears, moving outward to help clear the sinus area.

G = "GUNKY" EYES AND NOSE

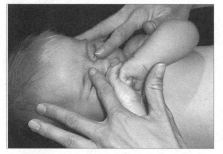

This is great for opening up clogged tear ducts and nasal passages.

Gunky Eye

- Many babies have "sticky eyes" when they are born, where their tear ducts may have been clogged. Using massage is a wonderful way to relieve the closing of the tear ducts.

- Gently place your fingertip in the corner of your baby's eye.

- Press in and rotate your finger in a circular motion, moving ever so slowly down onto the bone of the nose and then up again.

- Repeat this two to three times.

Gunky Nose

- Sinuses are little pockets that can get filled and cause discomfort.

- Take your index fingers and place in the corner of your baby's eyes, along the nasal bone. Press in and up, and glide down along the bridge of the nose from the top to the bottom.

- Repeat two to three times.

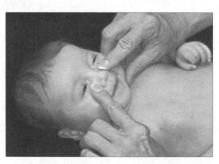

Your baby's sinuses under his eyes may also be blocked.

H = HI! I SEE YOUR SMILE

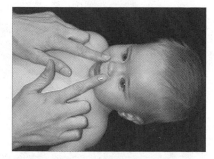

Smile and your baby will smile back to you.

- Start from the middle of the lip and end with tracing a happy smile.

- Make an outline of your baby's upper lip, stroking with both index fingertips.

- Continue to outline lower lips.

- You can sing this rhyme:

  Two little lips
  Are just like this
  I love you so much,
  Give me a kiss!

  (Here is a perfect time for you to pucker your own lips and give your baby a great big kiss!)

J = JEWEL DELIGHT

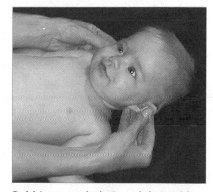

Rubbing your baby's earlobes adds comfort at the end of the massage.

- Gently rub the earlobes simultaneously with your index fingers and thumbs starting from the top, down.

- Rub the lower part of the earlobes.

- Cover the opening into the ear with your index finger as you rub.

- Some babies may not like having their ears rubbed. Many nerve cells are located in the earlobes. Check for any aversive reaction or other physical difficulties, and notify your baby's healthcare provider, should this persist.

K = KEEPING IT ALL TOGETHER

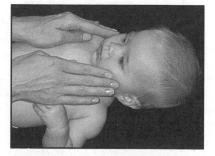

Ending the massage movements in unity will increase awareness of your baby's face and all body parts from face down to legs.

- Move your fingertips rhythmically outward and downward from your baby's ears to his chin.

- Hold your baby's face again in the palms of both hands.

- Let your stroke glide over your baby's face, down his neck, and down the whole body.

- This stroke unifies your baby by bringing all of the body parts together, preparing him for the next transition.

Newborn Strokes

Newborns are such "sleep machines" that their worlds are vastly different from the world of a baby who is two, three, or four months old. A newborn, sleeping eighteen hours or more each day, is processing information about his world even during his sleep. A baby who is two months old may sleep several hours less and begin reaching out and exploring his world, while a four to six month old is becoming more sociable.

When you are gazing at or holding your newborn, you may be ready to give your baby a massage, but is your baby ready to receive one? Your newborn may weigh seven or eight pounds and be twenty inches long, and you may think, "Can I even massage him at all?" The answer to this question is *yes*, you can massage your newborn, adapting the basic massage strokes to meet your newborn's needs—and your own.

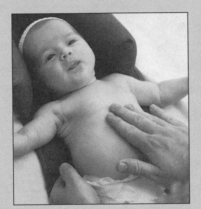

It is crucial that you watch and listen for those times when your newborn baby is receptive and quietly alert for massage. Also, since your newborn will have just recently begun using his own energy to breathe, digest, and maintain body temperature, you may choose to massage your newborn over his clothing if he becomes cold when his clothing is removed. You may swaddle your newborn to inhibit limb movement and provide constant touch stimulation (just like being in the womb), removing one body part from the swaddling at a time. You may use soft pillows and make a little "nest" for your newborn so he feels secure and protected.

Newborns need extra special care. For many, the umbilical cord stump may still be attached to the body—for up to two weeks or even four weeks of age. If you choose to massage your newborn with his umbilical cord stump on, avoid the area around or near it, as you must be careful to keep the cord stump clean and free from oil. Some of you may prefer waiting until after your baby's umbilical cord stump has fallen off before giving a massage with oil. Some of you may choose to gently stroke, hold, or pat your newborn over his clothing. Whichever manner you choose, you will be learning as much about your newborn as he will be learning about you. You will read your baby's cues and gain permission to massage, no matter how subtle your baby's feedback. Make sure you don't over-stimulate him as you A (Attune), B (Breathe), and C (Communicate), in A (Acknowledgment), W (Wonderment), and E (Enjoyment).

Your newborn's circuitry is growing and you are helping to structure his brain with your interaction. Dr. Candace B. Pert states in *Molecules of Emotion* that touching and hugging releases neuropeptides of pleasure and well-being. How much you interact and the quality of your interaction will show how much you care and will create lasting memories for both of you. So take a few minutes to read the following guidelines and massage your newborn with Dr. Elaine's TouchTime FLAIR.

Dr. Elaine's TouchTime FLAIR for Newborn Strokes

Frequency—You may wonder how often to massage your newborn during the day. You might stroke your baby each time you lift him up from his crib and put him over your shoulder. You may find yourself naturally rubbing his back as you soothe him or comfort him. While holding him, you may rub his arm or leg. You may gently pat his bottom as you cradle him in your arms. As your baby gets older, you may find yourself routinely massaging your baby once a day or several times a week, following the suggestions given in Chapters 3 and 5.

Level of quiet alertness—Newborns sleep a lot and are up for feedings, diaper changes, and sponge baths or bathing. Massage ideally occurs when your baby is in a *quiet alert state*. There may be little time for any alertness at this stage of growth and development. For now, you may find the time to massage your little one may be during the time your baby is awake and being held over your shoulder, or during a diaper change as part of your everyday routine. You may massage him without clothing using natural fragrance free oil or gently stroke him through his clothing without oil.

Amount—Since your newborn will sleep so much during the first month, you may find yourself shortening the time you thought you would spend stroking him. Don't be surprised if the full body massage is not tolerated just yet. Just introduce a stroke, and follow your newborn's cues to continue or stop. (Remember to keep one hand touching your baby when you reach for your massage oil.) Usually as your baby gets older he will be able to endure longer massage time periods. As your newborn becomes comfortable with your stroking one body part, you may introduce another body part slowly. Even massaging one or two areas is extremely beneficial for your baby and yourself, bringing relaxation to both of you while assisting in regulating your baby's bodily systems, such as digestion, elimination, respiration, and circulation.

Intensity—Newborns appear to be so fragile, and they are. Using your full palm for any TouchTime stroke movement may result in too much stimulation or too much pressure for him. Use one or two finger pads, rather than your entire hand, to gently and firmly stroke your newborn. I remember holding my grandnephew Corey in his little "onesie" with his chest against my chest and his face on my shoulder. While he was awake, I used just one finger to make circles along the sides of his spinal column. He enjoyed this stroke and fell asleep in my arms. "Nana Michele" told me she calmed Corey and soothed him to sleep by massaging him with just two fingers on his temples (Temple Rubbings) and ears (Jewel Delight).

Rhythm—You need not move too quickly when you are stroking your newborn. Remember that your newborn is just experiencing the world outside the womb each day. Before, he was floating around in amniotic fluid. Now, your gentle and firm touch may be a slow and steady rhythm reminding him of the place he used to inhabit. This mutual rhythm will be helpful in allowing your newborn and yourself to connect and calm.

In due time, your newborn will grow into infancy, toddlerhood, and childhood, giving you permission to engage in massage for longer and longer time and with more and more body parts. The benefits of touch have been demonstrated for newborns as well as for older children. In fact, it is vital to connect and communicate through touch during these important first days and weeks of your baby's life. Have fun! Go slowly and remember to engage your baby with love and respect. Follow his cues, and your relationship will grow—just like him.

DR. ELAINE'S TOUCHTIME BABYOGA HARMONY EXERCISES

All of us enjoy the benefits of exercise, once we get our body to the gym or make an effort to participate in some sports activity or begin daily walking. Yoga exercise loosens and stretches muscles and joints, and increases your flexibility, strength, balance, and range of motion. What better time than now to get your infant onboard a gentle exercise program?

The previous series of massage stroke movements are designed to relax, tone, and integrate your baby. Starting at about three to four months of age, the following gentle exercises may be done with your baby when your baby's muscles are warm, usually after the massage. Make sure that your baby gives you permission to move his joints, hips, and shoulders. When stretching out the leg or arm, make sure you support the joint closest to the body, so if his leg is outstretched make sure you hold under his knee, or if his arm is outstretched, hold under his elbow. Keep your baby in alignment. Don't pull or push your baby to go further than he can. When you see that your baby is uncomfortable with a yoga harmony posture, change to another exercise. For example, if your baby doesn't like his arms or legs opening so wide, you can go back to those exercises another day, slowly increasing the width his arms or legs can open. DON'T ever force a yoga position. Read your baby's cues and follow your baby's lead to determine how many TouchTime Babyoga Harmony Exercises your baby will be able to enjoy. Remember Dr. Elaine's rule of thumb: "Be gentle, and when in doubt leave it out!"

Many dads enjoy these exercises with their babies, because dads often enjoy the fun and frolic kind of play. When the baby is young, before walking, oftentimes dads don't know what they can do to connect with their baby. These gentle exercises give dads the opportunity to interact with their babies, encouraging flexibility, muscle strengthening, play time, and relaxation. As your baby gets older, and is beginning to cruise, scoot backwards, or try to stand, these physical exercises are more fun for your baby also. Just as it was important to check with your baby's healthcare provider before engaging in massage, check with your baby's healthcare provider before engaging in these TouchTime Babyoga Harmony Exercises, too.

Dr. Elaine's Babyoga Harmony Strokes

Remember your **ABCs** in **AWE**.

D = DANCING DOVES

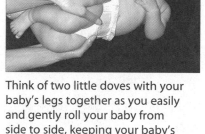

- Always align pelvis and back.

- Gently place your hands along the sides of your baby's torso and gently roll your baby from side to side.

- Repeat two to three times.

Think of two little doves with your baby's legs together as you easily and gently roll your baby from side to side, keeping your baby's spine straight.

E = EVERYTHING GOES

These are fun exercises that will encourage you to sing and rhyme as you go.

Pat-A-Cake

- Place your baby's hands together in front of him, palm to palm.

- Pat his hands together two to three times.

- Then gently hold your baby's hands and stretch his arms out wide at either side of the torso. Go as far as your baby is able, reaching out to find your baby's kinesphere. (How far can your baby stretch? Will he allow you to open his hands? Is he still protecting his hands and keeping them close to his body as he did in the womb? Gradually your baby will allow you to move his hands further and further apart. If he resists this now, go slowly. Read your baby's cues.)

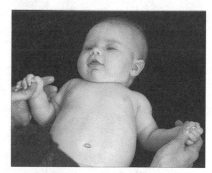

Gently stretch a little each time and don't ever force your baby's arms apart.

- Repeat this sequence two to three times.

- You may want to recite:

    Pat, Pat, Pat

    Open so W–I–D–E. (Hold the word "wide.")

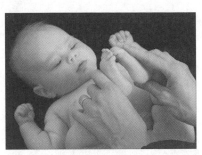

Pat-A-Foot movement

Pat-A-Foot

- Gently place your baby's feet together in front of him, sole to sole.

- Pat his feet together two to three times.

- You may want to recite:

     Pat, Pat, Pat
     Look at that!
     Pat, Pat, Pat and
     Rat-a-tat-tat.

- Repeat two to three times.

Jumping Jacks

- Reach one arm down to touch the opposite foot, as the foot is lifted up towards your baby's tummy.

- Hold for about three to five seconds.

- Move the leg and arm back to the beginning position.

- Reach the opposite arm to touch the opposite foot.

- Hold for about three to five seconds.

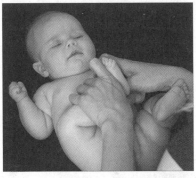

Jumping Jacks movement

Bicycle Built for Two

This is a fun exercise that will encourage you to sing and rhyme as you go.

- Bend your baby's knees gently, supporting your baby's legs under his knees.

- Move one knee toward the chest, and then the other one.

- Keep feet in alignment with knees and hips so your baby's hips do not rotate out or put any strain on your baby's knees.

- Continue alternating knees and pedaling while singing a song:

     Riding a bicycle all day long
     Riding a bicycle singing a song
     Riding a bicycle I love you so
     Riding a bicycle let's go, go, go!

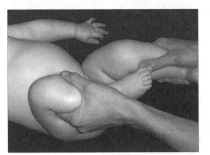

Bicycle movement

F = FOR OLDER BABY

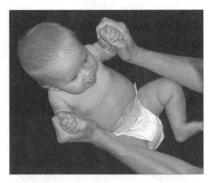

Sit Ups

- This is usually best to do if your baby is about six to seven months old or older.

- As your baby has been lying on his back for a while, you may hold onto his arms and see if he wants to get up from that position.

Sit Ups movement

Stand Ups

- This is for babies approximately eight to ten months old.

- From the sit up, if your baby is able, you can bring him into a standing position as you continue to hold his hands.

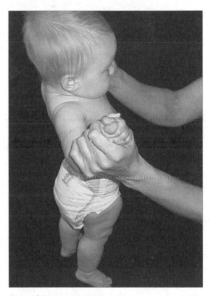

Airplane Ride

- All babies love to go high in a parent's arms.

- Hold baby with one arm under his stomach and hold his buttocks with your other hand, suspending him in the air with his stomach facing down.

- Hold him like an airplane gliding in the sky.

	or

- Hold baby with both hands under his armpits and around his midriff with each thumb on his chest and palms on his back while suspending him in the air.

Stand Ups movement

- Lift him up and down.

- "Fly" for five to ten seconds and watch him laugh and giggle.

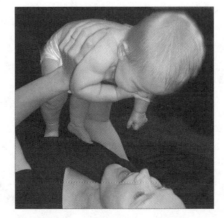

Airplane Ride movement

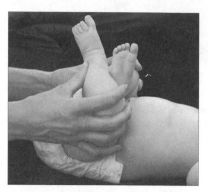

Gently bend and support baby's knees while crossing one leg over the other.

F = FLOWERING LOTUS

- Gently cross one leg over the other leg with one leg on the bottom and one leg on the top. (Be careful to keep your baby's legs underneath so that the hips are not thrown out of joint.)

- Switch legs so the opposite leg goes on the bottom and the other leg crosses over on top.

- Hold for a count of approximately five seconds.

G = GENTLE STRETCHES AND EMBRACES

Gentle Stretches

- Gently take your baby's legs and stretch them out from his torso.

- Hold for three to five seconds.

Gentle Embraces

- Hold your baby's wrists and stretch his arms out at shoulder height away from his body.

- Cross the arms at the chest, folding one arm on top of the other. This will release tension in the shoulders and upper back.

- Then release the arms by extending each one out to the side.

- Cross over the chest again, placing the arm that was on top of the other now on the bottom.

- Alternate the arms two to three times.

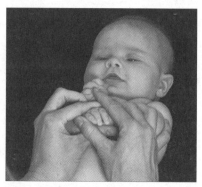

Crossing one arm over the other is fun.

Stretching baby's legs from the torso will make your baby feel "so tall."

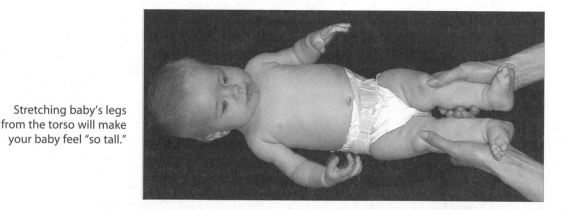

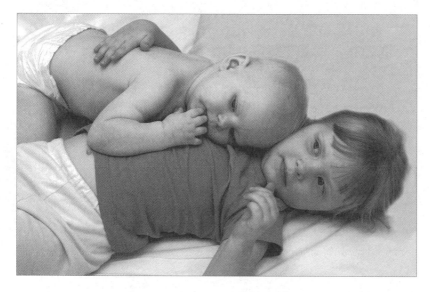

These two sisters hold each other close right after sharing their mommy and daddy in TouchTime massage.

H = HUGS, KISSES, CUDDLES, AND PRAISES

Mom tells her little girl just how wonderful she is and how blessed she is to have her.

Now it's your turn to:

- Hold your baby.

- Hug your baby.

- Kiss your baby.

- Cuddle with your baby.

- Sing your baby's praises.

- Say, "I love you!" and

- "I will love you forever!"

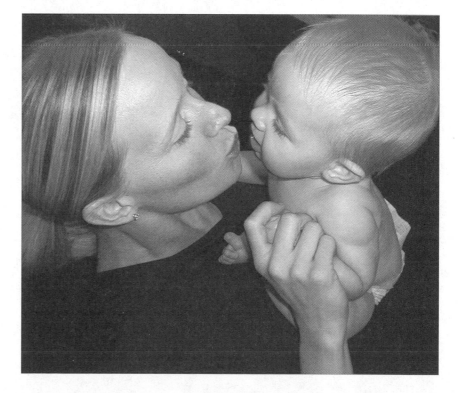

Let your baby be the leader in your massage encounters. Read his cues to determine if he is ready for a massage, and if he is comfortable and willing to partake in Dr. Elaine's TouchTime Baby Massage and Babyoga Harmony Exercises with you. You must be receptive to his needs and any changeable behavior. Never force a massage. Always check for contraindications. Keep massage sacred so that it becomes an important part of your daily rituals and routines. Remember that your dialogue, through touch, will provide the opportunity to enrich relationships that are forming now in these formative years, and will evolve into a two-way dialogue that will continue over a lifetime.

CHAPTER 4

SONGS AND RHYMES— USING YOUR VOICE TO HARMONIZE AND SYNCHRONIZE

Now that you know the ABCs of baby massage and the relationship that massage builds with your baby, you needn't be surprised to discover that baby massage is not just a time for using the sense of touch. If you have ever had a massage, it may be hard to picture your masseuse singing to you or rhyming words as you are being massaged, but with baby massage that is just what the doctor ordered! Your baby is developing physically, emotionally, and spiritually, and brain growth is vital during these early years. So your masseuse may not sing and rhyme to you, but as you massage your baby you will find the joy of belting out a song or rhyme with your baby's full attention. You will be providing the unique opportunity of attuning interactively while building neuron connections.

How many times have you held your inconsolable baby in your arms, only to start rocking her and softly singing to her so that she will go to sleep? How often have you noted that your baby calms through song and melody?

This chapter will explain the important aspects of using your voice in melody and rhymes in conjunction with baby massage, and the role music and rhymes play in your baby's awareness of the world around her. You will see how you can create simple little songs by using tunes that you already know. I have created a variety of songs and verses for parents that I will share with you so that you can use them, too. Remember, though, that just as every other aspect of baby massage requires that you read your baby's cues and follow your baby's lead, you will also need to be observant when using melody and rhymes. Make sure that the rhymes or music do not lead to over-stimulation, causing your baby to become disorganized, pull away or flail her arms, or show you any other signs of disengagement (see Chapter 2). If this occurs, reduce the amount of sensory input that is causing your baby's senses to become overloaded, and bring back rhythm, rhymes, and songs when your baby is able to accept them. Baby massage is a nurturing time for you and your baby. Enjoy the moments while creating lasting memories!

LISTENING INSIDE AND OUTSIDE THE WOMB

Babies are listening before they are born! The womb serves as a music hall, bouncing sounds in amniotic fluid with mom's rhythms as the harmonic backdrop for baby's life before birth. Your baby began to know rhythms and sounds as she was carried in mother's womb—the steady constancy of mother's heartbeat, the rhythm of mother's pace, and the sound of mother's and others' voices and everyday harmonics. Current research is discovering that the sounds your baby hears in the last trimester of pregnancy are recognized after birth. For example, according to DeCasper and Spence, the rhythm of the famous Dr. Seuss book, *The Cat In the Hat*, when read aloud to your fetus during the last trimester of pregnancy, will be recognized by your baby outside the womb shortly after birth.

Outside the womb, other amazing scientific discoveries reveal that a baby cries to the pitch of her mother's voice. When parents are talking and their baby is near, the baby's movements will move in the same rhythm of the parents' speech patterns. Brazelton, Tronick, and other child specialists have shown us how a baby can turn her head to pick out the voice of her parents from the voice of a stranger—moments after birth. So attuning to sounds is something your baby has been doing even before birth. Whether you were reading aloud, talking, or singing, your baby was hearing your voice and the voices of others.

LISTENING BEFORE BABY CAN TALK OR SING

Remember your ABCs (Attuning, Breathing, and Communicating) while experiencing the AWE (Acknowledgment, Wonderment, and Enjoyment) of massage. For a reminder, turn to pages 50 to 53.

In recent years, more researchers have been looking into the origins of musical capabilities than ever before. As a matter of fact, you can go to any baby store and find on the shelves compact discs for baby's listening. Did Bach or Mozart ever know they would be a household item for those who cannot even walk? Olsho's studies show that a baby as young as five months of age can tell the difference between the smallest tones between two notes. Infants eight to eleven months of age can remember and perceive melodic pitch changes, just like an adult. This has been demonstrated by Trehub, Bull, and Thorpe. Chunking words to help auditory memory also occurs when we group music into phrases. Rhythm and tempo, which are the building blocks for music, can also be detected by infants as young as seven to nine months of age. Weinberger has shown that the auditory cortex in the brain plays a role in detecting pitch, and it is this basic building block of music that is an important feature of brain organization.

Just as other studies have shown the dramatic abilities of newborns to remember a book they were read in their third trimester, we now have proof that babies can also remember tunes they heard. Hepper found that neonates two to four days of age, having heard a tune played to them while they were in utero, remembered that tune, as indicated by changes in movement and heart rate. Even more striking is that fetuses of twenty-nine to thirty-seven weeks (gestational age) also showed behavioral responses to tunes they were played earlier in pregnancy. Remembering melodies can occur before birth and before or at the beginning of the third trimester, as Weinberger states.

Infants have surprising capabilities just like adults, which allows us to look into our nature even more. Through massage, we learn that touch is not isolated from our other senses, and that when speaking it is not simply the words that matter. Through massage, we get to see the whole picture of communication. We learn about the closeness of our body; the quality of our hands' movement on our baby's soft skin; the cadence, harmony, pitch, and inflection of our voices; the smell of our body; our eye gaze; and the kinesthetic impressions our baby receives through our own movement/touch signature. This intermingling creates the messages we send and the messages our baby receives.

IT IS THE PERSON SINGING, NOT THE SONG

In addition to touch, your voice is a natural way of attuning with your baby. Each one of us has a natural signature we carry in our touch and movement patterns. We also have a natural signature we carry in our vocalization. Just like understanding the ABCs of baby massage brings you greater confidence in parenting your baby, when you realize the important ways that rhythms and songs enrich the relationship you have with your baby, you can throw away any fears or doubts of how you sound.

What does your baby hear when you sing to her? Do you think she listens to critique which sound is high and which one is low? Which one is fast and which one is slow? Does she care if you can hit a high note or can't reach one at all?

If you are like me, you can remember your mom singing to you or reciting nursery rhymes. I never had a thought about how good or bad my mother could sing; I just knew we were enjoying the melody together. It

Through massage, we learn that touch is not isolated from our other senses, and that when speaking it is not simply the words that matter.

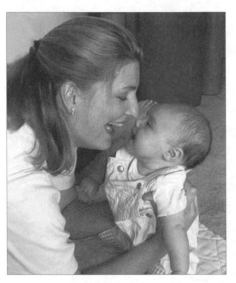

Mom and baby are harmonizing through mom's touch, rhythm, words, and voice. A key to baby massage is the inclusion of non-verbal and verbal dialogues.

wasn't until years later that I came to understand why I had such a good time when my mother sang to me. Learning all about brain growth and development, bonding, synchrony, and language development, I realized how important music, rhymes, and rhythms were for my own growth and development, and how enjoyable being with my "vocal" parent was for both of us.

The key to baby massage is the dialogue. In being close together, you and your baby bond and form a relationship to last over time. By exposing your baby to your voice, you continue to find more ways you can harmonize and synchronize and, according to Manolson, "help your baby make sense of the world, not tune out."

When you use your voice to include rhythm, rhymes, and songs, your baby's development is increased threefold. First, you are increasing her listening skills and auditory perceptual skills as your baby listens to your words, and as you match the words with your actions (such as "going up the legs"). Second, by including melody and language, you are fostering your baby's right and left brain growth (as described in Chapter 1). You are furthering language development by increasing vocabulary (such as, "Are you ready for your massage?"). You are encouraging social-emotional well-being by enhancing self-image (telling her "your leg is so soft and beautiful") and socialization.

This blending of voice and touch brings forth three languages: the language of touch, the language of words, and the language of melody. It is vital that we speak to our babies and allow them the opportunity to hear as much language and speech as they can prior to their own talking. We must remember that even when your baby cannot talk with words, she is like a little sponge, absorbing all that you offer.

Just because your baby doesn't speak in words doesn't mean that she cannot hear. Unless your baby has been diagnosed with a hearing disorder, your baby will hear, and learn the language system of her own family. Researchers have shown how important the first five years of life are for language acquisition. We learned from Noam Chomsky, expert MIT linguist, how babies are "prewired for language." When it comes to speech production, Flohr, Mehler, Spence, DeCasper and others affirm that newborns prefer the sound of their mother's voice over the sound of a female stranger, and their mother's native language to a foreign language.

Now we are learning that the biological roots of music are strong, too. And the best part is that your baby really doesn't care how you sound when you sing. She doesn't care if you can reach a high note or not. Your baby is just so happy to hear your voice, bonding and attaching through melody. You don't have to be the next Pavarotti, Celine Dion, Alan Jackson, or Kelly Clarkson to use melody and rhymes while massaging your baby and forming a loving relationship.

LETTING GO

The passing down of songs and rhymes from one generation to another may be lost when new parents live so far from their own parents. Often, it is the new parents who have to begin new rituals. Baby massage is one such ritual—as is singing and rhyming while massaging. I remember a father of twins I was seeing in the Baby Steps early intervention program. I was demonstrating infant massage and explaining the importance of also singing to children, of getting down on their level and engaging with babies within the massage—even if he felt like he was acting "silly." He couldn't quite understand how he was to behave. In his eyes, his twins didn't need to hear him talk, sing, or rhyme since they wouldn't talk, sing, or rhyme back to him. He said, "Singing and talking to my baby feels so silly. You expect me to act silly?" I said, "Yes." I explained to him that what he thought was "silly" was, in addition to touch and massage, a way that he could actively interact with his babies.

If you can talk, you can rhyme. If you can rhyme, you can sing.

So many parents feel that singing songs to their infants who cannot sing back is downright foolish. Other parents have told me that they don't know how to act babyish, and that they don't know how to sing. Some have told me that they are not very creative and don't know how to make up rhymes. If you can sing by yourself in the shower, you can certainly sing to your baby. It is really simple. Remove your ego from singing or rhyming and your self-consciousness will go away. How can you possibly feel self-conscious around your infant? What judgment could a two month old make? If you can talk, you can rhyme, and if you can rhyme, you can sing. Your baby is not evaluating your singing voice. Your baby is happy being together with you.

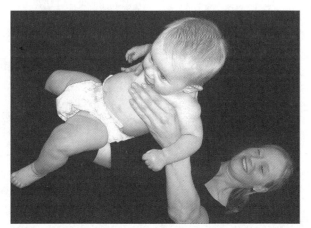

Mom certainly knows how to be creative and engage her baby in song and rhyme while propelling her daughter up into the sky. Baby is happy being together with mom and mom is happy being with her baby.

So, massaging your baby is not touching your baby only. More than one sense is working when you are massaging—touch, sight, hearing, feeling, moving, and smelling. You are joining together in a "dance." Let your rhythm move you and move your baby. You will be pleased how much your baby delightfully responds with widening eyes, or giggles, or coos to your melody and rhymes. When you are massaging your baby, you may find that you do not need or want to sing with each and every part you massage. You may find delight in singing, rhyming, or using your voice while you are massaging some particular body part. Begin with touch, and add words, rhymes, and non-verbal cues. Each is interrelated. Remember that adding songs and rhythms means more stimulation, so make sure that, as mentioned before, you read your baby's cues. If your baby shows signs of wanting to take a break from your extra input, then follow her lead. Remove the songs and see if she wants to continue, or take a cuddle break and return to massage later. You know best.

LETTING YOUR IMAGINATION SOAR

How can you make up songs and rhymes? So many parents tell me that they are unable to sing and can't make up any songs or rhymes on their own. They don't see their creativity. Others tell me that, at first, they had a hard time trying to make up rhymes or using songs and rhymes they already knew, but that with time they became more self-confident. They realized that if their baby smiled and cooed and giggled when they heard them singing or making up rhymes, the reward of their infant's smiling face was all that they needed to keep them inspired and keep them going. Then they could unwind and just let their imagination soar. Gradually they began to enjoy adapting rhymes and songs while massaging their baby. Parents who thought they didn't have a creative bone in their body began using their imagination, and learned that they had more creativity than they knew.

A person's voice naturally changes when talking to a baby. This high pitched, upward inflecting voice pattern is known as "parentese."

Language is not learned in a social vacuum. Who among you hasn't had the moment when, face to face with your baby, you lovingly started talking in a higher-than-normal pitch with simple words or sentences? I spoke about this "parentese" in Chapter 2. By the time your child turns four years of age, the level of your child's vocabulary and language development will be determined by the amount of language that your child has heard throughout each day.

Viewing the way babies develop, no matter what you do throughout the day, it is important that you talk to your babies. Massaging your baby provides the perfect time to rhyme or sing, capturing your infant's attention and maintaining communication. Each one of us has an imagination of our own, but often being "too busy" or feeling "too embarrassed" reduces this playfulness. Many parents have told me that changing diapers, feeding their baby throughout the day, or just being sleep deprived is not conducive to any creativity for song and rhyme development.

For those parents and caregivers that would like to have ready-made verses and rhymes to use, I have put together some rhymes you can recite or sing as you massage your baby's different body parts. In most cases, you can make up your own rhythm to the words I have designed for you. Other songs and rhymes are used from existing, common rhymes and songs, to which you can add new words. Regardless of the songs you choose, it is most important to remember massaging your baby is a time for you to be together. Adding your voice and rhythm provides more opportunity for furthering brain development, while having fun!

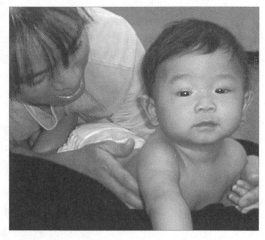

This mom enjoys singing a gentle lullaby with her baby.

SOUNDING OUT

In Chapter 1, you learned just how remarkable your baby's brain is. The division of labor between the left "language" brain hemisphere and the right "music" hemisphere shows how the brain has discernable organization that is intimately musical. Babies' love of music has strong biological roots. The musical infant is the normal human infant, possessing the capabilities of perceiving and mentally organizing music. Parents are the first music teachers a child has, and the bonding experience of listening together is as important as the type of music chosen. Here are some highlights of interesting information about sound and your baby.

This dad has no trouble singing and playing with his son. They are bonding through touch and rhythm.

- Babies hear by the eighteenth week of pregnancy, so bonding through sound occurs before birth.

- During the last two months of pregnancy, babies can hear both mother's and father's voice, music, and rhymes.

- Babies can remember verses recited to them while in the third trimester of pregnancy, and remember a melody before or at the beginning of the third trimester.

- Babies prefer music that mimics the mother's heart rate of sixty beats per minute, which is heard in the womb. Lullabies are good sources of this type of music.

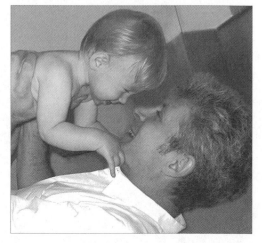

- Babies are sensitive to sounds of human speech.

- Babies can pick out the sound of their own parent's voices from strangers, moments after birth.

- Babies can distinguish between phonetic sounds like "ga" and "ba."

- Babies as young as four months old know the differences between melody and speech.

- Babies as young as four months of age know when the "Happy Birthday" song is played incorrectly.

- Babies seven to nine months of age can detect changes in rhythm.

- Rhythm and tempo are basic building blocks of music, and infants are able to perceive and mentally organize music.

- Animal studies show that constant exposure to chaotic music, such as heavy metal-type music, alters brain structure.

- Listening to music can improve the ability to perform complex tasks or spatial reasoning.

DR. ELAINE'S TOUCHTIME SONGS AND RHYMES FOR BABY MASSAGE

Now that you know the research information about the amazing relationship between sound and baby's brain, you can see the importance of music, rhythm, and voice for your baby. Here are many songs and rhymes that I have created for you to use while massaging your baby. Some of the verses may be sung to popular songs, while you may choose to use your own songs for other verses, when no specified tune is listed. Many of the rhymes and songs have a body part or a stroke movement in the title of the rhyme or song. Other songs and rhymes have emotions in the title. Select the ones you like. Each rhyme, song, and melody can be repeated as often as you choose. Let your voice be heard and let your own imagination soar, perhaps making up your own melodies that will become your own family tradition. And of course, if you would like, please send me copies of your rhymes so that they can be shared and added to the others I have received over the years.

Some of the following rhymes can be sung to popular songs, and I have listed the song after the title of the verse. Other rhymes can be simply recited. Unless a familiar tune is specified, feel free to create your own melody to the words I've written.

SONGS AND RHYMES FOR ATTUNING

Attuning with your baby sets the tone for your Dr. Elaine's TouchTime Baby Massage. These songs and rhymes encourage daily routines and rituals which will help bring your baby stability and consistency in an ever-changing world. These songs and rhymes will also bring you to a greater awareness as you slow down your own breathing, relax, and become alert and focused with your baby. Communicating with touch from your heart, respecting one another, and valuing the time you have together will enable learning and growth. Bringing your energy together, you form the bonds that lifetimes are built upon.

The following songs and rhymes will set the stage for a joyful baby massage and can be recited when you and your baby are attuning. Make up your own melodies if you'd like or just rhyme them. You'll find the Torso Touch and Energy Rolls massage stroke movements on pages 64 to 65. You may also note that the verse Rolling Along will appear in other sections of this chapter. That is because you may also like to use the verse when you are making circles on other body parts, like the top part of your baby's feet, using Happy Feet on page 69, or on your baby's back during Gentle Circles on page 83.

Attuning

Attuning with you
In my heart
Attuning with you
Is where we start

Energy Rolls All Day Long

Roll em roll em roll em roll em
Circles all day long
Roll em roll em roll em roll em
I love to sing our song

Rolling Along

Circles, circles everywhere
In our hands how much we care
Circles left and circles right
Being with you is such a delight

Respect One Another

Into the heart
Into the heart
Can't you see?
Let's just be
Respecting one another
Happily

Torso Touch

(Sing to *If You're Happy and You Know It.*)

Breathe in breathe out
Torso touch
Breathe in breathe out
Don't be rushed
Torso touch
Torso touch
We are ready torso touch
Breathe in breathe out
Torso touch

SONGS AND RHYMES FOR MASSAGING BABY'S LEGS

Your baby's legs are located just as far from her face as they can be. Many babies may feel less threatened when touched on their legs. Newborn babies' legs do not appear straight. Don't be surprised if your baby appears as if she just got off from riding a horse, as her legs are certain to be bowed. When your baby was in utero her legs were tucked up against her tummy and so often her legs will stay in that fetal position. You may gently stretch them down only to find them to rebound back into the tummy tuck position. Gradually they will relax and lengthen.

Your baby may enjoy having her legs massaged before other body parts. I like to start massage on baby's left leg and foot and when finished move to baby's right leg and foot. See which leg is comfortable for you and your baby.

The following melodies can be recited when you massage your baby's legs. See pages 65 to 71 for the various stroke movements to use on baby's legs. Several of the following rhymes may be sung to popular songs, while you may choose to make your own songs for the other verses, when no specified song is listed. Other verses may be interchanged during the massage. For example, *Knead, Knead, Knead* and *Squeeze and Glide* can be recited during the massage for legs, and they can also be recited during the massages for arms on pages 73 to 75.

This Is the Way We Go Down Your Leg

(Sing to the tune of *This Is The Way We Wash Our Clothes.*)

This is the way we go down your leg
Go down your leg
Go down your leg
This is the way we go down your leg
So early in the morning (*or you can say* late in the evening)

This is the way we squeeze your leg
Squeeze your leg
Squeeze your leg
This is the way we squeeze your leg
So early in the morning (*or* late in the evening)

This is the way we massage your foot
Massage your foot
Massage your foot
This is the way we massage your foot
So early in the morning (*or* late in the evening)

Down We Go

Down, down, down we go
From your hip down to your toes!

Knead, Knead, Knead

Knead, knead, knead
Watch you lead, lead, lead
Knead, knead, knead
Watch you lead!

Squeeze and Glide

Squeeze and glide,
Squeeze and glide,
Let's not hide
When you squeeze and glide

Reading your cues,
I learn the don'ts and do's,
Reading your cues
I learn the don'ts and do's

Rolling Along

Circles, circles everywhere
On your feet
How much we care
Circles left and circles right
Being with you is such a delight!

SONGS AND RHYMES FOR MASSAGING BABY'S BOTTOM OF FEET, TOES, AND TOP OF FEET

Your baby's toes and feet may be so busy every day, kicking in the air, at blankets, or at mobiles, or exercising their own movement pattern. Feet are like roots from which trees grow and which house energy. Stroke your fingers along the bottom of your baby's foot and until she is nine months to one year of age, her toes will fan out and her foot will twist inward in reflex. We know that energy exists throughout our entire body, yet according to the practice of reflexology, dating back 5,000 years, energy starts in the feet, with pathways leading to different parts of the body. So when you massage your baby's feet, by stroking, rolling, pressing, or rotating, it's as if you're massaging your baby's internal organs, glands, and muscles.

Remember some babies may have experienced heel pricks during their hospital stay. In these instances your touch may awaken your baby's "muscle memory" and may lead to aversion, withdrawal, and discomfort. You may need to hold her foot and gradually introduce massage as she becomes able to tolerate your touch.

Rolling each toe individually is so much fun as you rhyme or sing a song. Parents have told me that they never realized the importance of each little toe. Each toe grows bigger and bigger, providing a bigger base upon which to stand, walk, and eventually run. Also, differentiating the toes, one by one, increases flexibility and your baby's body awareness.

The top of your baby's foot is often covered by socks—how often do you get to touch your baby's soft skin on the top of her foot? It is important to massage the area that connects your baby's toes to your baby's ankle. Massaging over your baby's foot is a wonderful way to reduce tension, gain awareness of that body part, and prepare your baby for standing. With twenty-six bones in the foot, and so many muscles and nerve endings, it is important to massage both top and bottom, sending information to the rest of your baby's body and brain.

The next songs and rhymes go well when your massage takes you to the bottom of your baby's feet, toes, and top of the foot. Verses may be interchanged with massaging other body parts. For example, *Walk And Talk* may also be used when "walking and talking" across your baby's tummy using the Daddy Longlegs stroke movement on page 79. *Look At Me* may be used with any other stroke movements and body parts. You may like to recite *Piggies, Piggies, Piggies, Happy Little Feet*, and *Pretty Little Feet* when you massage your baby's toes. *Making Circles As We Go, Rolling Along*, and *Pretty Little Feet* you may recite as you massage the top of your baby's feet.

FOR MASSAGING BOTTOM OF FEET

Walk And Talk

(Sing to the tune of *Row, Row, Row Your Boat*.)

Walk, walk, walk, and walk
My fingers know the way
Walk, walk, walk, and walk
We can talk all day!

Look At Me

Look, look,
Look at me
Having so much fun
With (*Insert mommy or daddy, or the name of the person who is massaging*)
Look, look,
Look at you
Massaging is what
We love to do

FOR MASSAGING BABY'S TOES

Piggies, Piggies, Piggies

Piggies, piggies, one, two, three
Piggies, piggies, as cute as can be
Piggies, piggies, four and five
Piggies, piggies, a perfect size

Happy Little Feet

Happy, happy little feet
Little feet are really sweet
With five pretty little toes
They will surely, surely grow
1–2–3–4–5

Pretty Little Feet

(Parents love to kiss the sweet feet of babies.)

Pretty little feet
You are so sweet
Pretty little feet
What a precious treat

Rolling Along

Circles, circles everywhere
On the top of your foot
How much we care
Circles left and circles right
Being with you is such a delight!

FOR MASSAGING TOP OF FEET

Making Circles As We Go

Over the foot, over the foot
Isn't this cute,
We're over the foot
Making circles as we go
Making circles
High and low
Making circles as we go
Making circles
High and low

Rolling Along

Circles, circles everywhere
On the top of your foot
How much we care
Circles left and circles right
Being with you is such a delight!

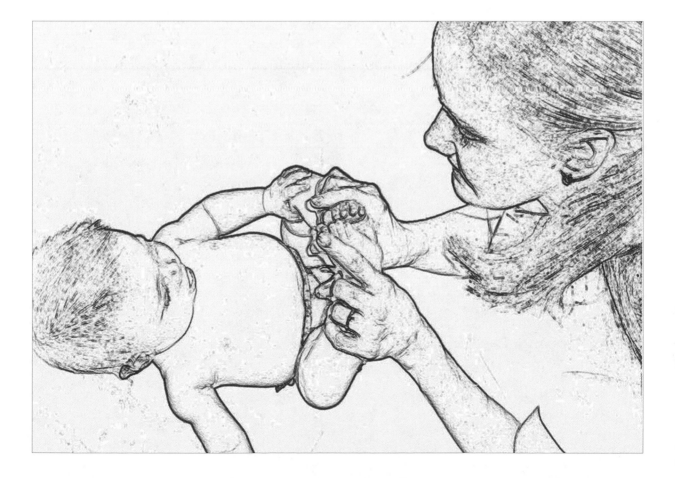

SONG AND RHYMES FOR MASSAGING FROM THE ANKLE BACK UP TO THE HIP

It's important to stroke back up from the ankle in the direction of the heart, after you have stroked away from it. Stroking towards the heart is more invigorating than stroking down away from the heart, which is generally more relaxing. This stroke sends the blood back to the heart and increases the venous flow. Like adults, babies develop tension in their bodies as they try to repeat actions they have just learned. It is so important to move the blood back up to the heart to help stimulate the circulatory system and bring balance to your baby's body and mind.

You'll find strokes for massaging your baby's leg from her ankles back up to her hip on pages 69 to 70. The following rhymes are perfect for this massage as you include the gliding stroke movement of I'm Moving Up which is found on page 69, and the pressing stroke movement of Joyful Touch which is found on page 70. You can also substitute the word "arm" for "leg" using these same rhymes when you are ready to massage from your baby's wrist back up to her shoulder on pages 74 to 75.

I'm Moving Up the Leg

I'm moving up the leg
I'm moving up the leg
Having so much fun
I'm moving up the leg

I'm moving up the leg
I'm moving up the leg

Having so much fun
My day has just begun

Back up the leg
I press, press, press
Back up the leg
Who'd want anything less?

Gently Up Your Leg We Go

(Sing to the tune of *Mary Had a Little Lamb.*)

Gently up your leg we go,
Leg we go, leg we go
Gently up your leg we go
And around your hip

Stroking it a little more
Little more
Little more
Stroking it a little more
Enjoy the trip!

Back Up the Leg

Back up the leg, with a jelly roll
Back up the leg,
We roll, roll, roll

Relaxing is Fun

(This rhyme goes great with Joyful Touch, which is found on page 70 and page 75.)

Feeling so easy
Is so much fun
Warm and flowing
Like the big, big sun

Feeling so easy
Is really great
So warm and flowing
A joyful state

SONGS AND RHYMES FOR MASSAGING THE SIDES OF THE TORSO

The Earth was discovered not to be flat, and neither are we! We have a front, a back, and sides to our body. From my training as a dancer, I know how important it is to integrate the entire body, whether big or small, and now you do too!

Babies' growth follows a pattern from the top down and the center out. So your baby's body grows from the center and moves outward toward the extremities. The sequence looks familiar when you realize that a baby will move her entire hand before she can control individual fingers. This sequence of growth whereby the growth begins at the center of the body and moves outward into the arms and then hands and legs and then feet is called the proximodistal pattern. Just like a tree standing tall, rooted into the ground with branches growing from the trunk, with massage your baby will sense the connection between her torso and her hips, legs, ankles, and feet, and her torso and her chest, shoulders, arms, wrists, and hands. She will gain self-awareness and body awareness, which are paramount for her growth and development.

These songs and rhymes were created just for your baby and you. The massage stroke Darling Baby appears on page 71.

My Darling Baby

My darling baby
My precious baby
I love you more
Than you'll ever know
Let's stay together
Let's play together
Till _____ comes home (*insert the name of a family member*)

Darling Baby

Darling Baby
You're full of charm
From your feet
Up to your arms

Darling Baby, Too

Darling Baby, Darling Baby
You're so sweet

From your arms
Down to your feet

My Sidekick

(Sing to the tune of *London Bridge Is Falling Down*.)

You have feelings in your side
In your side, in your side
You have feelings in your side
My dear baby

Take my hands and
Glide up, up, up
Up, up, up
Up, up, up

I take my hands and
Glide up, up, up
My dear baby

SONGS AND RHYMES FOR MASSAGING BABY'S ARMS, HANDS, AND FINGERS

No matter how many songs and rhymes I've written, parents always keep asking me to write more. Here are some for massaging your baby's arms, hands, and fingers. Sometimes when you begin massaging your baby you may find her hands held tightly against her side, or her little fists may be tightly shut. Remember that in the confines of mother's womb, she could not stretch her arms too far, nor could her hands reach out in space. Probably as far as her hand may have reached was with her thumb reaching right to her mouth as she sucked it. Babies also have a natural grasping reflex (Palmar grasp). This reflex usually weakens after three months, is usually outgrown by five to six months, and disappears by one year of age. So do not be surprised if your baby makes a fist when her palms or fingers are touched.

From the time your baby is two months, she can hold a rattle briefly, transferring one object to another at about five months of age. At seven-and-a-half to eight-and-a-half months, your baby can grasp with her thumb and her finger, and by eleven or twelve months she is putting three or more objects in a container.

You have the privilege of massaging your baby's extremities, which are vital for holding and reaching, not just for your hand or your fingers, but for everyday functions such as holding a bottle, or a finger food, and eventually buttoning a jacket or shirt. Baby explorations are also possible when arms enjoy a range of motion and hands have dexterity to hold a rattle, reach out for a mobile, or touch a leaf for the very first time.

Following are some songs and rhymes for massaging your baby's arms, hands, and fingers. Enjoy these rhymes and songs. Make up your own verses. You'll find these massage stroke movements on pages 73 to 75.

Going Down Your Arm

Going down your arm
Going down your arm
Don't be alarmed
I'm just going down your arm

Rubbing as we go,
Rubbing as we go,
Get into the flow
We're rubbing as we go

Up from the wrist
Up from the wrist
We move up from the wrist
And then you are kissed

Relaxed little arm
Relaxed little arm
So full of charm
You're a relaxed little arm

Round and Round We Go

(Sing to the tune of *London Bridge Is Falling Down*.)

Take your wrist and turn it so
Turn it so
Turn it so
Take your wrist and turn it so
My fair lady (*or* gentleman)

Take your wrist, don't let it go
Don't let it go, don't let it go
Take your wrist, don't let it go
My fair lady (*or* gentleman)

Gently Up Your Arm We Go

(Sing to the tune of *London Bridge Is Falling Down*.)

Gently up your arm we go,
Arm we go, arm we go
Gently up your arm we go
And across your chest

Holding it a little more
A little more
A little more
Holding it a little more
You're the best

Down into your fingertips
Fingertips
Fingertips
Down into your fingertips
To reach the world

Circles, circles in the air
In the air
In the air
Circles, circles in the air
My special dear

Around your wrists I do go
I do go
I do go
Around your wrists I do go
My sweet baby

Back to your heart
To your heart
To your heart
Back up to your heart
My sweet baby

Five Little Fingers to Keep Me Happy

Five little fingers to keep me happy
I have five little fingers to keep me happy
1–2–3–4–5

SONGS AND RHYMES FOR MASSAGING BABY'S CHEST

The chest houses many organs, including your baby's heart and lungs. Your baby experiences life through movement. The word "emotion" comes from the root word "emote," meaning to release through movement. As you massage this part of your baby, as mentioned in Chapter 3, you may find your baby letting go of sounds as if she were telling you a story. Listen and watch empathetically and allow your baby to "vent." You may find yourself not singing a song or rhyming, as your baby communicates, and you listen to her. Or you may find yourself massaging your baby's chest for a while longer than anticipated so she can have the time to fully express herself.

Research has shown that even when two different heart muscles are severed and continue to pump in separate Petrie dishes, the two separated hearts will synchronize to one another and begin beating in unison. Think about this as you massage your infants and toddlers. You know the old saying, "one heart feels the other," and this is certainly true both figuratively and literally. Your baby's lungs are also housed in the chest, which are vital for your baby's breath. As stated in Chapter 3, breathing is important as a life source, and proper breathing will enable your baby to go FAR—becoming Focused, Alert, and Relaxed. (You will too!)

The following songs and rhymes can be recited when you are massaging your baby's chest. *Dear Heart* can be used with the Dear Heart baby massage stroke movement on page 76 and *Fancy Circles* can be sung to your baby when you are using the Fancy Circles baby massage stroke movement on page 77.

You Are the Very Best

(Sing to the tune of *Row, Row, Row Your Boat*.)

Smooth, smooth, smooth your skin
Gently on your chest
Merrily, merrily, merrily, merrily
You are the very best!

Across, across, across your chest
Spread your wings so wide
Across, across, across your chest
Let me be your guide

One heart
Two hearts
Three hearts
Four
I love you so much
One heart
Two hearts
Three hearts
Four
So tender to my touch

Dear Heart

Dear Heart
I love you
And it is really true
For as long
As I'm living
Dear Heart
I love you

Engaging Wings

Criss-crossing your chest
Criss-crossing your chest
You're at your best
When I'm criss-crossing your chest

Rolling Along

Circles, circles everywhere
On your chest
How much we care
Circles left and circle right
Being with you is such a delight!

Fancy Circles

Fancy circles on your chest
Going east and going west
You're the one
I love the best
Fancy circles on your chest

SONGS AND RHYMES FOR MASSAGING BABY'S TUMMY

You learn a lot about digestion when you have babies because one of the major conversations you will have is about "pooping." Diapers, bowel movements, and constipation are just part of everyday conversations.

On a physiological level, when you massage your baby's tummy you are not massaging her stomach. Rather, you are massaging the part of her body that covers her intestines, which are responsible for moving waste products in a clockwise motion out of your baby's body. Her stomach is actually up towards the left side of her body, nearer to her heart and tucked up under the ribs. When your baby is constipated, massaging the tummy has significant benefits as your action aids the movement of waste products through her intestines.

Always massage clockwise so as not to "back up her plumbing."

Some Eastern medicine practitioners say that the tummy is also another place that houses strong emotions, and so massaging this area can help soothe your baby as she has another opportunity to express herself. Be gentle and read her cues. Use the following melodies when you massage your baby's tummy. Strokes for massaging the tummy are listed on pages 79 to 80. The rhyme *For Fun Galore* may be recited with the Fun Galore—Legs Up High and Fun Galore—Legs Down Low stroke movements on pages 79 to 80. Gentle Breezes can be used with the stroke of the same name, and the rhyme *Round and Round We Go* may be used with the Earth Watch stroke movement on page 79.

Tummy Time

(Sing to the tune of *London Bridge Is Falling Down*.)

Across your tummy we will go
We will go
We will go
Across your tummy we will go
My fair baby
Round and round like _____
    (*Insert* a steering wheel *or* the morning sun)
A Steering wheel (*or* The morning sun)
A Steering wheel (*or* The morning sun)
Round and round like a steering wheel
    (*or* the morning sun)
My fair baby

Down the tummy we will go
We will go
We will go
Down the tummy we will go
My fair baby

Down your tummy
With your feet up high
Feet up high
Feet up high
Down your tummy
With your feet up high
My fair baby

Round And Round We Go

Round and round we go
Like the morning sun
Round and round we go
Our fun has just begun

Crossing Your Tummy

(Insert your baby's name in the space below.)

_____ is a big, big honey
He's/She's letting daddy/mommy/
    nana/etc.
Cross his/her tummy

Get the bubbles out, out, out
Get the bubbles out, out, out
And then we all will be happy

For Fun Galore—Legs Down Low and Legs Up High

Put your feet low
How low can you go?
Put your feet up—so high
Put your feet up to the sky

Gentle Breezes

("Gentle Breezes" is explained on page 80.)

Oh the ease of a gentle breeze
Calling my name so softly
Come with me, I'll go with you
And we will be so happy

Rolling Along

Circles, circles everywhere
On your tummy
How much we care
Circles left and circle right
Being with you is such a delight

SONGS AND RHYMES FOR MASSAGING BABY'S BACK AND NECK

Your baby's neck and back are holders of much tension. You may ask how a baby can have tension when they look so flexible. Well, just think about your baby's large head. How difficult is it for your baby to hold it up? Have you noticed that it wobbles from side to side until approximately fourteen weeks of age? Then she can hold her head steady for short periods. It is not until approximately twenty-seven weeks that she can consistently hold her head up without it falling back. Sometimes it may take you nearly six months to find your baby's neck at all, hidden among the layers of baby's dimply skin.

We all know how calming a back massage can be. All the nerves of your body enter the spinal cord at some level. Just think of your baby laying on her back, or being held in a carrier or sling with her back against the upholstered fabric or a stiff carrier. Backs are a source of tension and benefit from massage. Stroke your baby's back up from her buttocks to her heart to stimulate her, and stroke down her back to relax her. The following rhymes can be recited when you massage your baby's back and neck. *Fanning the Fire* can be used with the stroke movement Fanning the Fire (page 83) when massaging your baby's back. *Heavenly Wings* may be used when you use the Heavenly Wings massage on page 83. The remainder of the stroke movements are on pages 82 to 84.

Fanning The Fire

(Sing to the tune of *Open, Shut Them.*)

Easy gliding, easy gliding
Right down to your feet, feet, feet
Fan the fire, fan the fire
It is such a treat, treat, treat

Circle circle, circle, circle
Near your spine, spine, spine
Crossing over, crossing over
How truly divine (*You can stretch out the word D–I–V–I–N–E*)

Gentle breezes, gentle breezes
Right down to your feet, feet, feet
Gentle breezes, gentle breezes
It is such a treat, treat, treat

Circle, circle, circle, circle
Near your spine, spine, spine
Crossing over, crossing over
Everything is fine (*You can stretch out the word F–I–N–E*)

How Divine

(Sing to the tune of *Twinkle, Twinkle, Little Star.*)

Circles, circles around the spine
How I wonder how divine
To the left and to the right
Oh my, what a beautiful sight

Circles, circles around the spine
How I wonder how divine
To the left and to the right
Oh my, what a beautiful sight

Easy Wind

Wind, blowing over
Wind, blowing over
Like a kite up in the air
Wind blowing over
Wind blowing over
I'm so glad you're here

Flying

My neck loves you
My shoulders too
I will tell you why
When you touch me with your hands
I just want to fly, and fly, and fly

Rolling Along

Circles, circles everywhere
On your back
What do we care?
Circles left and circle right
Being with you is such a delight!

Heavenly Wings

Criss-crossing your back
Criss-crossing your back
Look at that
I'm criss-crossing your back

Criss-crossing your back
Criss-crossing your back
Look at that
I'm criss-crossing your back

SONGS AND RHYMES FOR MASSAGING BABY'S FACE

All of the bodily senses are housed in your baby's head. That's right, along with her skin, which is the largest organ of her entire body, her other sense receptors are either on the front of her face—eyes, nose, mouth; or on the side of her face—ears; or inside her face—proprioception and kinesthetic receptors. The face is a carrier of lots of information.

Your baby spends so much time feeding, crying, and smiling as she gets older, that her face may also become a source of tension, just like her legs, neck, and back. Sometimes your baby may be reluctant to receive a facial massage as she may feel uncomfortable with touch on this delicate structure that was the first body part to emerge into the world of sights, sounds, and temperature. Also caution is needed when-

ever you touch the scalp, as your baby's fonatels (soft spots) are still growing. (The back fonatel usually closes at about four months of age, while the front fonatel may close between nine and eighteen months.) You may decide to massage your baby's face, and not her scalp, until her fonatels close.

There is nothing quite as wonderful as looking into your baby's eyes and seeing your beautiful baby, a little angel, looking back at you. This reciprocal gaze is just one manifestation of how you fall in love with your baby and she in love with you. Try reciting these verses when you massage your baby's face. Turn to pages 86 to 89 for these massage stroke movements and remember that you don't need to use any baby oil when you massage your baby's face.

Bright Eyes

Your eyes so bright
Morning to night
What a beautiful sight
Your eyes so bright

Gently, gently, down your nose
Gently, gently, like a pretty rose

Smile out smile out
See what I've been missing
Smile out smile out
Your lips so sweet for kissing

Angel Face

The face of an angel
Looks at me
The face of an angel
I love what I see
You were sent from heaven
So special and divine
You were sent from heaven
So glad you're mine

Beautiful Girl, Beautiful Boy

(Sing to the tune of *You Are My Sunshine*.)

You are my little _____ (*insert* girl *or* boy)
My little baby _____ (*insert* girl *or* boy)
You are so beautiful
In every way
I love you so much
I love you so much
When we **touch**
both night and day

(Replace the word **touch** with other words to create more verses to this song. For example, sing the entire song again and replace the word **touch** with another word such as **kiss** . . .)

When we **kiss**
Both night and day

When we **sing**
Both night and day

When we **hug**
Both night and day

When we **dance**
Both night and day

SONGS AND RHYMES FOR DR. ELAINE'S TOUCHTIME BABYOGA HARMONY EXERCISES

These exercises are playful, enjoyable, and gentle. They combine yoga stretches with playful parenting. Just remember, don't overstretch your baby's limbs; keep your baby's spine aligned; and keep your baby's knees in line with her hips. Babies need to stretch and reduce tensions held in their limbs, torso, face, hips, and neck, just like adults do.

Through these exercises your baby will be able to keep her body harmonized, deepen her own breathing, reduce stresses, and balance her mind, body, and spirit. A flexible body with a flexible mind creates an opportunity for harmony and growth. Remember to read your baby's cues and just like you would never force a massage, never force Babyoga. In time your baby will come to enjoy the exercises if she doesn't enjoy them at first. These exercises are especially important to do when your baby's limbs and muscles are warmed up. Have fun. Read your baby's cues and you will decide the frequency and duration of these Dr. Elaine's TouchTime Babyoga Harmony Exercises.

The following songs work well when recited with the TouchTime Babyoga Harmony Exercises that appear on pages 93 to 97. Some of the rhymes and songs are written for specific Babyoga exercises.

Happy, Happy Hearts

(Sing to the tune of *Bicycle Built for Two.*)

Happy, happy all day long
Happy, happy singing a song
Happy, happy our hearts so true
Happy, happy I love you

Legs crossing over
One and two
Legs crossing over
How do you do?

Looking At Me

Looking at you, looking at me
I'm as grateful as I can be
Looking at you, looking at me
This is perfect harmony

Looking at you, looking at me
We are so happy
Looking at you, looking at me
We are one big loving family

Love

Universal rhythm
Unconditional love
Our energies connect
With one another
Right from the source

Massaging and holding
You as only I do
No one knows better
How much
I love you!

All Through The Town

(Sing to the tune of *The Wheels on the Bus,* with the exercises for Everything Goes found on pages 93 to 94.)

Your two strong arms go open and shut
Open and shut
Open and shut
Your two strong arms go open and shut
All through the town

The soles of your feet go tap, tap, tap
Tap, tap, tap
Tap, tap, tap
The soles of your feet go tap, tap, tap
All through the town

Your arm and leg go up and down
Up and down
Up and down
Your arm and your leg go up and down
All through the town

Look At You, Look At Me

(This verse can be used with the strokes for Everything Goes, part of the yoga harmony exercises found on pages 93 to 94.)

Look at you
Look at me
We are s—o—o—o—o
H—a—a—a—p—p—y

Stretch your arms
Stretch your arms wide
Stretch your arms across
And don't be surprised

Do a pat-a-cake
Do a pat-a-cake
Roll those hands
And shake, shake, shake

Wrist and ankle
To the opposite side
Hold them gently
Then open them wide

Pedaling All Day Long

(This verse can be sung with the Bicycle Built for Two yoga harmony exercise found on page 94.)

Pedaling, pedaling
All day long
Pedaling, pedaling
With this song
Pedaling, pedaling
Isn't it great?
Pedaling, pedaling
We won't be late!

Flowering Lotus

(This verse is named for the stroke Flowering Lotus found on page 96.)

Do the legs cross
Do the legs cross
Cross over the tummy with a gentle
    and firm touch
Do the legs cross
Do the legs cross
Cross over the tummy
And don't be in a rush

Do the legs cross
Do the legs cross
Cross over the tummy
With a gentle and firm touch
Cross over the tummy
And don't be in a rush

One knee bent up
The other out straight

One knee bent
Now isn't this great?
Switch your legs over and
Don't be late

One knee bent
The other out straight
One knee bent
Now isn't this great?

Music is a way into the soul. It certainly opens up our relationships with one another as we laugh and sing together. Look around and you will hear the natural rhythms of life: the sound of a bird flying and squawking overhead; the sound of the ocean waves; and the sounds of the human voice. Kuhl shows that infants from birth to four months of age are "universal linguists." They can distinguish each of the one hundred and fifty sounds of human speech. By the time your baby is six months of age, she can distinguish the sounds of her native language. At eight to nine months of age, your baby's understanding of spoken words (comprehension) outweighs her ability to say the words (expression) she hears. Vital for your baby's brain growth and development is that she hears words and is exposed to them. Children exposed to greater vocabularies will develop larger vocabularies, resulting in higher IQs than those children who were not exposed. The music that structures your baby's brain is equally vital.

I hope you enjoyed these rhymes and short refrains. In no time, you will be making up your own rhymes, songs, and melodies. You have the power to start family rituals while having fun. You will also be creating lasting memories. There is nothing that you can't imagine in your songs. Don't let your ego get in the way. Let the words come from your heart. Express yourself and enjoy yourselves.

CHAPTER 5

$\mathcal{D}$IFFERENT AGES— WHAT TO EXPECT

You are never too old for a massage! When you begin the family ritual of massage with your child as an infant, you needn't be surprised to find the tradition you have established with your baby carries on into childhood, teenage years (yes, teenage years), and adulthood. The connections that were rooted early in infancy continue to grow throughout the lifetime of your relationship. And if you are just starting to offer massage to older children, it's never too late to relate!

In this chapter, I will share basic information about the benefits of massaging an older child. I will provide various heartfelt stories that both parents and children have shared with me over the years. I will share photos showing how massage is vital for healthier, happier, and more relaxed children—at any age.

MOVING ALONG WITH MASSAGE

Often parents will tell me how they were able to massage their babies when they were infants, but as soon as their babies started crawling, baby's intense desire to seek out the world took over. No longer could the parent find that quiet alert time for the massage, for it seemed that their baby was on *active alert* all the time! As babies grow, they gain strength in their necks, arms, and legs; their head is able to lift upright; they turn over; and they creep backward and forward, gaining so much more mobility to explore their world. Lying quietly on a mat or on a fluffy quilted bed may be wishful thinking when the baby has at his disposal his "all fours," which allows him to move anytime and anywhere he chooses. Ah, independence! You look forward to the time when your baby will grow and become more independent, and then you realize how much more control you had when your baby was dependent on you to move him from place to place.

This change in mobility certainly alters massage opportunities, but not necessarily for the worse. Parents, grandparents, and other adults who care for babies and children on a daily basis (including day care providers) have asked me, "Dr. Elaine, what can I do when I want to massage my child but he is so active now, crawling all over the place?" I have told them not to be concerned. Massaging your older child does not always look the same. Be attuned to your child; he will show you or tell you (when old enough to make formal requests) when the time is right to engage.

As stated in Chapter 3, massages do not need to be long, intensive experiences. There are many ways to massage toddlers, older children, and even teenagers that have the benefits of the earlier massage—improving health, happiness, and calmness while promoting bonding and closeness. Massaging feet, hands, sore backs, and making games out of massage strokes (like "flipping a pancake") are ways you and your older children will relate.

CHANGING STROKES FOR CHANGING BODIES

Remember your **ABCs** while experiencing the **AWE** of massage. For a reminder, turn to pages 50 to 53.

As your baby grows from infancy to toddlerhood and into childhood, the number of bones stays the same, as do the number of muscles. However, the length of the strokes you use and the quality of the strokes may change. Your baby's ability to tolerate more pressure may allow you to change the firmness of your strokes, adding a little more pressure to each stroke. Also, the speed and pressure of your stroke may be increased, introducing strokes that look like you are dicing onions or knocking on a solid oak door.

Your baby's growing bones and muscles will require that you use longer strokes for massaging longer legs, arms, backs, or necks. A more active child may tolerate an abbreviated massage rather than a full massage. Also, an older child usually tolerates fewer massages throughout the week instead of the daily ones that you may have been able to get in with your infant. Children who are beginning to crawl and move on all fours may still enjoy their massage, but it begins to look different. Staring up at mommy or daddy is not the most interesting position to be in when you can turn yourself over and begin crawling away on your own.

In your child's next developmental stage, which I call the "explorer stage," you will use your attuning and reading cues abilities to the max, figuring out where and how much massage your child desires. For some children, massage after bath time will still be wonderful, a time during which you continue bonding and relating as before. For your baby who is sitting up on his own, instead of massaging him after the bath, you may find that now you can massage him inside the bath. As you are swishing the soap bubbles around, I bet you are already making "Engaging Wings" and "Fancy Circles" and other strokes too, but perhaps just never called and recognized them by those names.

As your child gets older, you may also find that massage may be done through clothing without any oil at all. With children as young as two years old, you will also find that with their increasing verbal abilities comes their ability to let you know when they want a massage by asking for one, and even more specifically which body part they want massaged. I am reminded of little Edgar who, at twenty-six months, was able to tell his mother to rub his feet and that he didn't want any oil! Other children may still find it delightful to be fully massaged using all of the strokes after bath time and before falling asleep. But we have to realize that our child has likes and dislikes just like anyone else.

As your child grows, he will be able to voice the kind of massage he likes and dislikes, when he wants to be massaged, where he wants to be massaged, how, and by whom. Just like us, he will develop his own preferences. As caring parents, we always want to remember that our parenting role includes being responsive to our child's needs, being flexible, and honoring our child's uniqueness. We don't want to be so rigid in our thinking as to believe that every massage has to look the same.

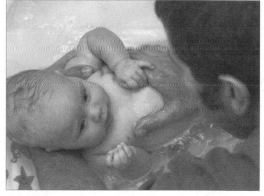

Baby and dad frolicking in the bath with Engaging Wings.

The key to remember is that TouchTime Baby Massage is a time for you to be with your child, reading your child's cues and developing harmony and closeness. The length of time you are able to engage in massage is not important. Being together and offering nurturing touch, of any length, is reassuring to your child, offering him the security he needs as he grows and explores his world. Whatever stroke your child may enjoy, continue your reciprocal relationship of giving and receiving, while following your child's lead.

Even though the massage moments you provide will be different at various stages of your child's growth and development, the same six principles still hold true: Attune, Breathe, and Communicate in Acknowledgment, Wonderment, and Enjoyment.

The chart on page 128 is for you to see the differences between massaging your baby and massaging your child. However, remember that this is a general chart. You are the best reader of your child's cues and would be best served by following your child's lead. Use the strokes that you know your child enjoys. Have fun being together. Communicate through touch, and always get permission before and during your massage.

With each of your infant's experiences, new and tremendous brain growth is occurring. You will want to take tender care to make sure that the room (where a massage will occur) is warm and that you follow the guidelines in preparing for a massage as listed in Chapter 2. As your baby

DR. ELAINE'S GUIDE FOR MASSAGING BABIES AND CHILDREN

Massaging Your Baby	Massaging Your Child
ABCs	ABCs
AWE	AWE
Read your baby's cues	Read your child's cues
Get permission before massage	Get permission before massage
Get permission during massage	Get permission during massage
Your baby is non-verbal	Your child is verbal and can ask for a massage
You observe your baby and decide the areas to massage	Your child can tell you what body part he wants massaged
Follow your baby's lead	Follow your child's lead
Remove clothing for a massage	Respect your child's decision for clothing to be on or off
The environment is prepared for massage	Your child tells you his environment of choice
Use a gentle and firm touch	Increase firmness, as tolerated
Use one stroke per body part	Use two strokes per lengthened body part. (Divide the stroke at a joint area, i.e., stroke from the shoulder to the elbow then from the elbow to the fingertips or from the hip to the knee and from the knee to the toes)
Start with one or two fingers moving into full hand with strokes	Use full hand or fingers with strokes
Use easy sustaining strokes that are slow and steady	Use quick and "chopping" strokes, in addition to slow and steady strokes
Hand stays on body	Add stroke flicking off body at end of massage (as if brushing away breadcrumbs from your lap)
Sing a song, make up a rhyme, or describe the body part you are massaging to increase body awareness	Create stories that go along with strokes ("a thunderstorm with pounding rain" or the "waves of the ocean gently breaking against the shore" while massaging your child's back) to foster creativity and enjoyment

continues growing from three to six months, he is exploring. At about six to nine months, your baby is finding out more about sitting and rolling over. You may add more songs and rhymes and even introduce a musical instrument for your baby to hold or watch so you can keep his attention as you massage him. From about nine months to one year, you may find that your massages are more abbreviated. You may massage in the bath or give a back massage before your baby goes off to sleep.

As your baby grows into toddlerhood, he may be just too busy for a massage, or you may find that adding lots of stories and games may keep him interested. You could also include some TouchTime Babyoga Harmony Exercises described in Chapter 3, and find that he enjoys being an airplane or moving his legs as if on his bicycle. When your baby turns three, you will find that he will be able to direct you into the type of massage that he likes. This is the time when your baby can tell you about his desires for his own body and what feels good. This can continue into your child's school-aged years and into young adulthood. Through touch, as you continue to grow your relationship with your child, the closeness that you felt at birth and infancy will continue to grow. School-aged children, teens, and young adults will always be "your baby," and turn to you for comforting. Be prepared to be there for your child throughout whatever age or stage he goes through, and in turn he will be there for you, too.

Just the other evening, I was sitting on the couch reading a book about a cosmetic entrepreneur when my daughter, who was studying for a law school entrance exam, sat down next to me on the couch. She placed her shoulder next to my shoulder. We never had to exchange any words as we sat together, touching one shoulder to another, and feeling that comfort and love as we connected.

FITTING MASSAGE INTO DAILY ROUTINES

Even when your older child seems to be more interested in activity and not in the quiet alert state for massage, you might find more time than you thought where massage would be a nice addition. You just need to start looking at different events during the day.

I have listed for you some of the times throughout the day during which you can include Dr. Elaine's TouchTime Baby Massage moments in your daily routines for the older child. Keep in mind, massage need not require a full half-hour or hour, where you lavish stroke after stroke with your child. Massage will take many different forms in many different environments. Hopefully your communication moments through touch will take only "seconds" and eventually become second nature to you and your child.

During Diaper Changing

Even though your toddler is able to either crawl or run away from you, until he is approximately three years of age, he will still need diaper changes. Keep some baby massage oil on the changing table or with your changing mat. As you change a diaper, you can massage your toddler's feet, hands, or legs. You don't need any oil to massage your toddler's face. Lovingly speak to your baby as you massage him, and sing a rhyme, letting your toddler learn more about himself while enjoying your time together.

During Story Time

During story time, when you have your little one sitting next to you or in your lap, and you are reading a book, you can gently rub his toes, hands, or even stroke his back or neck. Making the loving contact, acknowledging your little one's presence, and reading his cues will only bring you even closer during this special time together.

Before Leaving the House or Going off to School

So many times we wonder how our child will do when he leaves the house and goes off to school. We wish we could go with him, making sure he is safe throughout the day, but also know that doing that would not create independence in our child. One way that you can tell your child that you care, which only takes a short time (thirty seconds or a minute or two), is to place your hands on your child's back, with his permission, and give a little shoulder massage. Give him a pat on the back and tell him to have a good day. This feeling of being touched by a parent with words of encouragement will instill a sense of pride and well-being in your child, as he will know that someone cares about him.

Traveling in a Car or on a Plane

During an airplane or car ride, you may find your toddler becoming fussy, wanting to run and play. You know he would do anything to get out of his seatbelt and run down the aisle in the plane, or jump around in the car. Body parts such as the face, legs, and feet are readily accessible for you to massage, even in a plane or car. After asking permission, Steven's dad discovered he could massage his son's face, helping him relax and fall asleep on a cross-country plane ride. Steven said he preferred his face to be massaged by his dad's firm and gentle strokes (rather than his mother's), which helped him forget about his fear of flying, and relaxed him to sleep.

Sarah's mom discovered she could relax her daughter, reducing her need to get up and move around the car during a long seventy-mile drive from home to the city. By getting permission and then massaging Sarah's toes and doing the Going Dancing stroke on the bottom of her feet, Sarah relaxed and was able to stay in her car seat for the entire ride into town.

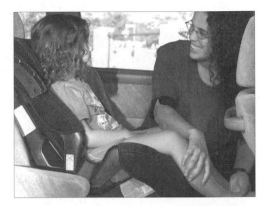

Massaging restless feet and legs in the car or van can make for a more pleasant ride.

At Bedtime

Hailey visited her grandmother often. She especially enjoyed sleeping over at her granny's house because when it was time to go to sleep, granny

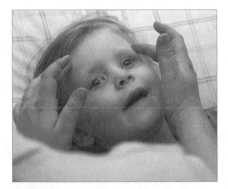

Hailey enjoys her very own Temple Footprints and granny says, "It doesn't get much better!"

would take her fingers and "draw little angel wings" on Hailey's' forehead and on her cheeks. Hailey loved the attention grandma was giving her, and she loved the special way she felt having those angel wings on her face. (Angel wings on Hailey's forehead are like Temple Footprints; angel wings on Hailey's cheeks are like Funny Faces Cheek Circles— High and Low in Chapter 3.) Now at five years of age, whenever she is with granny she asks for her "angel wings" to be "drawn on her face."

I know of two women in their thirties who remember a bedtime ritual with their own mothers. Mom would pull their long hair back away from their faces and place it over their ears before they went to sleep. To this day, that touch is so soothing to them that they still ask their mothers to pull back their hair when they visit one another.

Hailey knows that she is respected and appreciated and values the love she feels with her granny. She feels that the bond she and her grandmother have is unique and a special one that will not disappear in her lifetime. She values the security she feels having the regular massage routine provided by her granny. What's also great is, to find out how they feel about one another, just ask Hailey's granny. She will tell you, "It doesn't get much better."

After Sports or Recreation

As far back as I can remember, my daughter has played soccer. It seems that she played soccer as soon as she could walk and run with the smallest of children in our local AYSO leagues. As a high school student she played on her high school varsity team. She loved the sport, whether she scored goals or defended the net. After a game, I always remember her going into our house, sitting down on a couch in the family room and asking me, "Can you massage my feet? Ple-e-e-ease?" I remember the moments we shared talking about the game with her legs outstretched as I massaged her feet. She felt so much better after relieving the soreness of her feet, and getting into a stress-free zone. I felt good as a parent knowing that I was able to provide this stress reduction for my daughter, and an opportunity for her to share her feelings about the game with me as I massaged her. I also appreciated her wanting my hands to massage her and relieve her soreness. This interchange allowed us to share special moments, ensuring the continuance of our close relationship.

Whatever sport your child now plays or will play, and whatever other recreational activities your child may engage in—dancing, boating, camping, or marching in a band—following with massage can become a routine and part of your daily life. Your child can ask you, just like my daughter asked me, "Will you massage my feet? I'll do anything you ask if you massage them. Ple-e-e-ease." What power we parents hold in our hands!

In Day Care Settings

Parents are not the only people who take care of children and can benefit from knowing about massage. During the many presentations I have given, day care providers were intrigued to learn the role that massage could play in their setting, not just with babies, but with older children, too. After first obtaining parental permission, they appreciated adding massage to their daily routines. Getting a group of pre-schoolers to take a nap in the middle of the day is no easy trick when you are a day care provider. Children wander around the room, start crying and fussing, and require lots of energy on the part of the day care provider. Having even one child begin crying or wandering may set off the other children in the group.

By using massage when it is time for "their children" to lie down for a nap, day care professionals have a way of relaxing them through their own hands. This seems to ease the transition from "up time" to "down time." Learning about a child's likes and dislikes is a way for providers to become more in tune with a child in their care, and the benefits are enormous. Some of the day care workers I have spoken to have told me that they began noticing that babies in their care became fussy at the same time each day. So, several minutes before this fussiness usually occurred, the workers would engage in massage with the babies and watch how the babies calmed.

Ms. Arlene said that Jake, two-and-a-half years of age, would always rebel against taking a nap. Often you would see the group of pre-schoolers lying down on their cots, and Jake would be walking around the classroom. It wasn't until Ms. Arlene began massaging Jake's back before he lied down that she noted how his body began to relax under her touch. Now he takes his "blankie" to his cot and goes off to nap like the other kids, instead of walking around the room.

During Storytelling Time

This storytelling time is different from story time. In story time you massage your child as you are reading a book, reading a story. During storytelling time you are creating the story as you massage your child's body. You can usually do storytelling on a child's back, as that is the part that older children enjoy getting massaged, with their faces down, even with their clothing on. You can be as creative as you choose, making up your own story lines. Some parents describe ocean voyages, others tell about making a fajita, and still others may tell a story about a thunderstorm turning into a beautiful rainbow. I enjoy stories about nature, with hummingbirds and trees blowing in the breeze.

For a reminder of the ABCs of massage, turn to pages 66 to 67.

My husband used to tell our daughter stories about a girl named Karlotta (a fictitious name my husband made up that was close to our daughter's name). This girl lived in days gone by and would have many vast travels and adventures. He would describe her family and how she became a princess. To this day, twenty years later, our daughter still remembers those magical moments she spent on her father's lap, or in her bed listening to the stories her father told her.

If you think you need some help with storytelling while giving a massage, I will share a story I have made up, which you can use with your older child. As always, make sure that you have obtained permission for the massage, whether you asked permission or your child has directly asked for a massage. Make sure you are relaxed in your own way so that this moment you share is not tension filled, but one of true joy. Use the ABCs of massage—Attuning, Breathing, and Communicating.

As your child chooses the location (bedroom, family room, living room), he may lie face down on a surface of his choice (the floor, on a couch, on a bed), indicating he would like to have his back massaged.

Respecting your child's choice and modesty, which is a natural part of development, your child also gets to decide whether he will have his clothing on or off.

Massaging your older child is a time for your child to guide his own massage based upon his choice of what feels good to him. He can tell you if he wants his back massaged or maybe just his feet. Many times when storytelling is used, you will find that your child's back is an easy place to massage. Older children like their backs massaged since it is the least threatening of all body parts, the position is easy to get in, and they find that when their back becomes relaxed so does the rest of their body.

With your older child, begin the interchange as with the infant massage—respect, ask permission, and receive a "yes" response. Use strokes for the back that you have learned in Chapter 3. As previously explained, you may find yourself using longer strokes, or dividing limbs into two, such as the hip to the knee and the knee down to the foot.

You can start by stroking the back of your child from his neck down to the back of his knees and then to his ankles. As you massage, you begin to tell your story. Using your firm and gentle touch, you also use your firm and gentle voice. You need to make sure your child can hear what you are saying. You need to speak loud enough so he can hear your voice, but not too loud that your voice becomes overbearing.

Following is Dr. Elaine's TouchTime massage story, and corresponding massage strokes. Try reciting the story while performing the accompanying strokes on your child's back. You may stroke two to three times for each verse.

Dr. Elaine's TouchTime Massage Story	*Compatible Massage Stroke Movements*
One day as I was walking in the woods Walking so gently so as not to disrupt the deer, the woodpeckers or the rabbits	Stroke firmly and gently from neck down to the back of the knees and then from the back of the knees to the ankles and feet.
I came upon the beach and saw the waves caressing the shore Back and forth and back and forth	Stroke your hands back and forth moving across the back while moving down the back, one hand next to the other. Your fingertips on one hand move up towards the right arm while the other fingertips on the other hand move down towards the left arm (perpendicular to the back).
Little sand crabs were digging into the sand, making their own little homes where they could live	Place your hands on either side of the spine making circular motions, right hand going to the right, left hand going to the left.

Then I saw a sailboat far away
Criss-crossing the ocean to get
Closer to land

Take your hand from your child's hip and stroke up and across to the opposite shoulder. Repeat with other hand from hip to opposite shoulder.

While the breeze gently blew
The sails were getting lower
And lower

Use a brushing motion, allowing each hand to comb from the neck down to the buttocks and down to the feet.

Finding the way into land
The sailboat came to dock
And the sun set at the end of
A beautiful day

Light strokes are allowed with the older child as finishing strokes, stroking lighter and repeatedly with less weight, and even lighter until your hand is held suspended over your child's back and you continue to breathe in and out for about five to ten seconds.

The above strokes and story are rather soothing and calm. There will be some children who, as they get older, will like more forceful strokes, and ones that are more percussive, like the chopping action as if chopping vegetables. For these children you can have the wind blowing more vigorously. The story line can be changed so that a thunderstorm is brewing and you may have the boat trying to get to shore in choppy waves. The verse could be changed to look like this:

Dr. Elaine's TouchTime Massage Story

Compatible Massage Stroke Movements

While the breeze started blowing
A storm came up and
The waves got so choppy
Thrashing everything in sight

Make little fists with the edges of your hands and tap them along your child's back.
Or, you can use an open hand with thumbs up and use the edge of your hands (not the thumb side) to do little percussive strokes (like cutting vegetables) from the neck, down and across the back.

You will want to end the story in a calming fashion, so just continue the massage, changing the ending to say:

Dr. Elaine's TouchTime Massage Story

Compatible Massage Stroke Movements

Finding the way into land
The sailboat came to dock
And the sun set at the end of
A stormy day

Light strokes are allowed with the older child as finishing strokes, stroking lighter and repeatedly with less weight, and even lighter until your hand is held suspended over your child's back and you continue to breathe in and out with your hands suspended for about five to ten seconds.

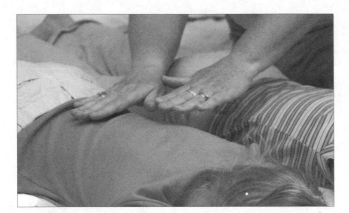

Here friends experience the closeness of one another, lying together as the sun sets at the end of a stormy day!

Combining a story with massage strokes fosters creativity in your child and yourself as you describe events in your child's life or you make up your own stories. So much fun and excitement occur as each child gets to go on a special trip, or dance among the stars, or experience the rainbow after a thunderstorm. You can always make up your own stories just like my husband made up his "Karlotta stories," which my daughter remembers to this day.

Throwing a Party

Many times we go about our daily routines and miss the opportunity of celebrating an event. So with older children you can actually put together a "household massage party" where everyone in the household sets aside a time during the week and brings his own oils or gels. (During the first ten to twelve months of life, I do not usually use scented oils. After that age, you can find out what scents your child likes, and have a trained aromatherapist prepare oils for you.) Throwing a party will work depending upon the participation of all of the family members. You can set up the amount of time you have for the party beforehand so that your older children will know that there is a beginning and an end to it. In our family, we would also hold a "sunshine party" where we would celebrate being outdoors in the sun and smooth on suntan lotion for each other.

Another type of party that my friend Susan told me about is one she calls the "couch potato massage party." You make a pact with your family that, along with sitting and watching television in the evening hours, during television commercials you give permission for your shoulders or head or arms to be massaged. As always, your child's willingness to engage in massage with you is paramount. Never force your child to participate. You can encourage, but not demand, when it comes to massage. Continue to follow your child's lead, honoring his wishes, likes, and dislikes. If he still says "no," then honor that and find another time and place and ask again.

READING THE CUES OF OLDER CHILDREN

I instructed Jeana in baby massage for her daughter Cassady. This extraordinary family consists of Jeana (mom), Brian (dad), Leah (Cassady's twin sister), and Jacob (three-and-a-half-year-old brother). Jeana had her hands full taking care of three children below the age of four, including Cassady, the twin with special needs. Brian worked all day and Jacob saw Cassady getting much attention from therapists and other physicians since her birth. What Jeana discovered about children and infant massage was what we know about three-and-a-half-year-olds—they observe everything and are very curious.

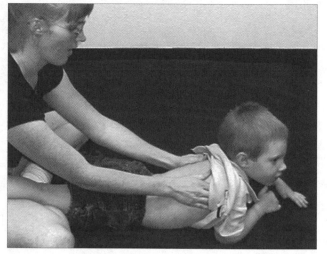

Jacob had seen his mom massaging Cassady, having their own special time together. One night Jacob, out of the clear blue, asked for a massage, too. Jeana said that she had always tried to relax her son as he "buzzed" through the house. Especially after bath time, she thought it would make him relax and go to sleep more easily. However, Jacob would never tolerate her massage after the bath, or before it for that matter. One day, after Jeana's infant massage instruction, I called her to see how things were going, and to see if she had any questions. She said that she was feeling confident massaging her daughter and becoming more flexible with scheduling the massage time throughout the day. She remembered to read her daughter's cues and follow her lead, and the massage time was becoming more and more special for both of them. Her voice became more excited, however, when she told me that not only was Cassady enjoying the massage. She said, "You won't believe it, but my three-and-a-half-year-old son is now asking for a massage before he goes to sleep."

Mom is told by her older son how he likes to be massaged; feeling confident and attuned, she follows his lead.

What was so wonderful for Jeana and Jacob was that Jeana did not have to coerce Jacob or bribe him. It was Jacob who spontaneously requested a massage. In her infant massage instruction, Jeana had learned about making sure to read her child's cues. With that skill she now learned that Jacob had a definite preference of how he liked being massaged. Rather than use oils to massage her son, which she had tried, she learned that Jacob enjoyed being massaged after his bath in his bed, right under his covers, with his pajamas already on. She learned that he preferred not having oil used on his skin before he went to sleep. She discovered that Jacob gained the benefits of massage through his clothing and he slept deeper and longer than ever before. Jeana had gained confidence in massaging her infant, only to discover that she was now able to massage her older child, too.

Older children can communicate their requests to you. Jacob gave

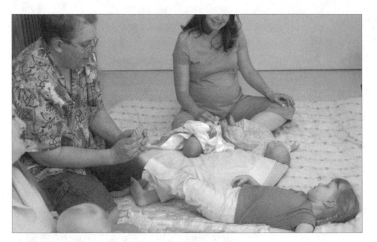

This little girl loves the attention her dad gives her, and dad is enjoying this special time together. These TouchTime moments help to grow relationships and are what memories are made of!

directions to his mom. She acknowledged his request, wondering where it would take them, only to find that their relationship deepened, increasing Jacob's physical well-being and her own, too! I'm sure that getting your child off to sleep, especially a deep one, brings you not only peaceful moments, but also peace of mind. All of this improves your health as well as that of your child.

Jacob's dad was able to massage Jacob with much enjoyment, too, as the whole family added massage routines to their daily schedule. I was so happy that the parents were able to find some time for all of their children, while also benefiting themselves.

THOSE PRE-TEEN AND TEEN YEARS

I remember hearing wise people say that when you meditate for twenty minutes, it is like getting more than an eight-hour night's sleep. I believe that by using nurturing touch with pre-teens or teens you can gain extra insight that may not come solely by using words to communicate. As a matter of fact, there are many parents who have shared exactly that discovery with me. They have told me that they knew something was wrong with their pre-adolescent or adolescent child. Maybe it is that sixth sense that people talk about when you feel that there is something unspoken standing between you and another person. They asked their child to tell

Dad's Coming Home from Work!

Hailey's dad had learned about infant massage when Hailey was younger. He never thought it would turn into so much fun when she got older, too. He enjoyed the time he could spend with his five-year-old daughter after he got home from work. This was his time to let go of the day and be with his daughter, and this was her time to be with her dad while her mom was making dinner. So many parents are so busy throughout the day that it is hard to truly connect with their children during the day or at night. Using massage allowed Hailey's dad to connect with his daughter. He massaged her back through her clothing. He massaged her arms, hands, head, and legs. When he was done he kissed her feet. How would you feel as his daughter? Would you feel special? Would you feel happy? Would you feel relaxed and calm? Would you feel secure? Would you feel loved? Hailey did!

Being Flexible Throughout the Day

Your TouchTime moments may vary from one stage of development to another and from one massage to another. One day your child may be as content as can be getting massaged after his bath. On another day, your child may want to receive a massage right after you get in from work to connect after being apart for the day. You may have one way of massaging and interacting with your baby when he is an infant and not crawling yet. This will change as he gets older. Don't get into a rut and think that massage has to look a certain way, or only be used at 7 PM every night.

Events occur, emotions vary, and needs change.

Be responsive to your child's requests, and massage moments may be initiated from your child as he gets older. Being sensitive to your child's needs, you may continue to initiate the massage by getting permission from your child. No matter who initiates the massage, the foundation of mutual respect and togetherness are the basic tenets of massage. Massage is an interchange between two people who are attuned to one another. As stated before, massage is a dialogue and not a monologue. No matter what you discover together during your massage time, remember flexibility.

them what was wrong. They tried to help the child, but he would not really open up and tell the parent what was on his mind. So the parent would read his cues.

Eventually, the parent was given permission to massage the child's back or shoulders, and while engaged in this stroking, the child opened up, letting the parent in and relating what had happened at school, or whatever was bothering him. The parents told me that massage then became one strategy they would use whenever they saw their child sulking or "closed." Many of these parents already had a history of using massage in their families, and turned to it to help bridge the gap between them and the older child. Building your relationship through touch can relax your child and allow him to speak—revealing inner feelings and hidden secrets that may not otherwise be available with words alone.

For example, Benjamin was not the most popular boy at school. He wasn't always picked for the sports teams. One day he had his heart broken because he thought that he would be selected for the varsity team. When he got home and walked through the door, his mother took one look at him and knew he had had some disappointment in his day. She asked him what was wrong, and he said, "Nothing." She asked him again, saying, "If nothing is wrong, why do you look so down?" Benjamin didn't answer. He went into his room and she followed. He sat on his bed, and she sat next to him. She touched his shoulder and he didn't flinch. She asked permission to rub his shoulders, and he didn't say no. Moving deeply into his shoulder muscle tissue, Benjamin broke the news that he

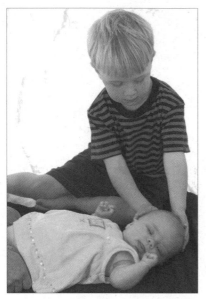

Big brother loves his baby sister and strokes her before mom begins her massage.

hadn't made the varsity team. Now mom had a way of dealing with her son's pain and disappointment, and he felt better being able to tell someone about how he was feeling.

GENERATION TO GENERATION AND SIBLING TO SIBLING

I am reminded of Lourdes, who told me at a presentation recently how, as a baby in the Philippines, her mother massaged her daily. When she had her children, she massaged them and now they are all grown up and married with their own children, whom they massage. Lourdes and her children have a close relationship, and she has a close relationship with her grandchildren—even though some of her family members live thousands of miles away.

When baby Eliyah was born, her brother Liam was already two years old. He had received massages from his mom, dad, and grandparents ever since his birth. It was natural for him to want to touch and massage his little sister, even though he could barely talk to tell you the difference between gliding and holding. But he knew how good it felt to be with his mom or dad or grandma and be the recipient of a massage. He is used to massage oil and having his own special family time. He felt included when he touched his sister's head at the beginning of her massage.

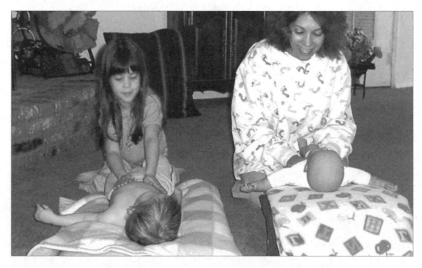

Big sister loves to be nurturing by massaging her brother. Dr. Elaine massages her own "baby."

Like Mother, Like Daughter

Lisa, now forty, told me she remembers the enjoyment, when she was younger, of receiving shoulder massages from her mother right before she went out the door to school. It was just a couple of minutes together when the two of them connected through touch, and the feeling of the massage carried Lisa throughout the day. Lisa's mother reported how years later, when she would come home from a hard day at work, her daughter would look at her and ask her if she had a long day and then offer to massage her weary shoulders. Now this massage carried Lisa's mom throughout her day and made her life all the more worthwhile.

The children who were once the "center of the universe" with no other siblings soon find themselves moving up the ladder of command in the family as births occur. Learning and using infant massage strokes and engaging in a meaningful relationship with their brother or sister is truly a blessing for both children. Since the "older child" was massaged as an infant himself, he will internally understand the principles and know the benefits from his own experience. Using infant massage in this way, to include older siblings along with nurturing parents, may be used as a relationship-building strategy.

Robby's five-year-old sister Michelle saw her mom massaging her brother and wanted to join in learning how to massage her brother too. Mom observed the interchange to ensure that she was careful and loving towards her baby brother and enjoyed being the big sister. Mom was happy that her daughter was learning this nurturing touch towards her brother and was developing their close relationship.

BENEFITS OF MASSAGE FOR THE GROWING CHILD

Many times older children are unaware of how to accept nurturing touch, how to say no to someone's touch that is inappropriate, how to relax their own bodies, and how to truly speak from their heart. Massage can help children with these issues.

Growing older need not separate us from our children. Finding ways to stay connected as we watch our children grow more independent and mature is part of the "heartstrings-pulling" that every parent feels. Many times when you begin massaging your older child, he can be transported back to the muscle memories of days gone by when he was relaxed under your touch when younger. The safety and security that your child feels allows him to reveal inner thoughts and cares that he may not have been able to describe in everyday life.

Similar to Benjamin's story, Rosemary told me about her own family story. Her daughter had come home from a Girl Scout meeting appearing to be distraught and sad. When Rosemary asked her why she was sad, eight-year-old Jennifer did not tell her, but said, "I'm not sad" and walked away. Later that evening when they were getting ready for bed, Rosemary's daughter asked her mom to rub her back. As her mother's warm and loving hands massaged her back, Jennifer relaxed under her mother's touch and told her mom that the Girl Scout leader did not select her to deliver the Girl Scout cookies. This "opening up" allowed Rosemary the opportunity to listen to her daughter, empathize with her, and tell Jennifer about a similar experience she had once had and the solutions she took that helped with the sadness she felt.

Another benefit of massaging your older child, besides being a channel for communication, is that massage provides him the opportunity to strengthen his physiology. With hormones raging during the pre-teen and teen years, your older child benefits by being able to relax himself, reduce his stress level, and seek out appropriate touch. As discussed in Chapter 1, there are many physiological and physical benefits to massaging your child. In addition, massage is a way for your older child to experience the following social-emotional benefits:

- Integrity as his wishes are honored

- Self-worth as measured by the time you share together

- Leading as he directs you

- Independence as he remains connected

- Continued bonding with the people who are so important to his own growth

- Relaxation and nurturing

- Appropriate touch

- Sensitivity from another

- Self-awareness

- Pleasure in a direct loving way

- Enjoyment with another

- Ability to say "no"

There are also many social-emotional benefits for parents. These include the opportunity to:

- Connect with your child

- Keep lines of communication open

- Further your sense of your ability to parent

- Enjoy your own relaxation and reduced blood pressure and heart rate

- Find a way to spend time with your child

- Respect your child's lead and honor his wishes

- Gain confidence in meeting the touch needs of your child

- Gain compassion for what your child may be going through in his own developmental stage

- Honor the time you have together

No matter what the age of your child, your relationship will always be important. Using TouchTime as your "SPECIAL TEACHER" will bring forth a healthy relationship that is:

S ecure	**T** rusting
P redictable	**E** nriched
E njoyable	**A** ttuned
C ommunicative	**C** aring
I nclusive	**H** appy
A ccepting	**E** ngaging
L oving	**R** espectful

WHAT YOU SOW YOU SHALL REAP

Older children enjoy giving back to their parents what they have been receiving. Older children have more strength in their legs and hands, and so when parents or grandparents are weary or need to be touched, their own children or grandchildren can be the ones to offer a loving hand. I know there were many times that I would get home from work and my daughter would see me dragging and say, "Mom, you need a massage. Let me rub your back." She did and I was forever grateful.

Many times when I provide infant massage classes to families, older siblings will attend with their parents, grandparents, or others. The sib-

Remember your ABCs (Attuning, Breathing, and Communicating) while experiencing the AWE (Acknowledgment, Wonderment, and Enjoyment) of massage. For a reminder, turn to pages 50 to 53.

lings are invited to come along, as are grandparents, day care providers, and others who are interested in learning about infant massage. Dolls are provided to those with no infants so they can practice learning the strokes. Usually children as young as three years of age are intrigued by watching massage, and will be willing to give you a massage, too. In fact, by about five or six years of age, children have the ability in their hands and "feet" to give a massage that feels good.

So many times your child will be agreeable to "walk on your back," "pound your shoulder blades" (how often does your child get to give you a good pounding, especially with you asking for one?), or just rub your hand. When you receive a massage from a child, often it is spontaneous. Your child may, in passing, see your needs and simply inquire, as in my family, "Can I massage you?" Or perhaps you are a family who enjoys making dates and so you and your child may make a special date to rub your back during your favorite television show (as mentioned in "Throwing a Party" on page 136). Now you can begin to see how worthwhile it was to give your own baby a massage, because now that he is older, he can return the favor.

Just as in infant massage, the same AWE of massage is in effect as you Acknowledge, Wonder, and Enjoy, while you utilize the ABCs of Attuning, Breathing, and Communicating. Many times parents tell me how much they enjoy having their backs massaged, or their hands and even their faces. Here are some simple ideas you can use so that your three-year-old child can massage your back. I've listed four additional ABCs for the older child—Ask permission, Be involved, Consider postures, and Select stroke movements—to remember how your older child can massage you. The additional ABCs on the following page work well for outlining how you can provide TouchTime massage for your older child, too.

Different strokes have different sounds or movements and can be enjoyable for your child and for you. It is really so simple. Kneading action, percussive movements, and stroking may be familiar to your child or remind him of things he has played with or heard before. For example, kneading your back may be similar to the way that he manipulates Play-Doh. Percussive movements can be like beating a drum. Stroking can be what he does with his pet cat or dog. Heavy touch may release stress and tension in your

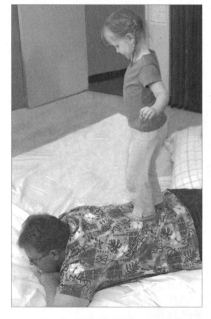

Dad considered the posture he would take on the floor while he and his daughter mutually selected the stroke movement, walking the tension right out of dad's back, in this joyful ritual.

ADDITIONAL ABC'S FOR DR. ELAINE'S TOUCHTIME MASSAGE FOR PARENTS BY OLDER CHILD (THREE YEARS OLD)	
Ask permission	As with infant massage, permission is always asked for and received. You may ask your child to give you a massage or your child may ask you if you want a massage.
Be involved	You and your child will have mutual respect for one another, knowing that massage time is not a time to hurt anyone, but rather a time to make someone feel better; a time to show caring and tenderness; and a time of acceptance, acknowledgment, and appreciation.
Consider postures	You get to choose which position works best for you.
	You may lie down on the floor, face down, or sit in a chair.
	Your youngster may sit or kneel on your back or stand.
Select stroke movements	Your child may choose the types of strokes he wants to give.
	You can ask your child for certain strokes and where you want the strokes.
	If you are lying on the floor, your child's weight on your buttocks can help your lower back release pressure and tension accumulated throughout the day.
	Your child may also massage your shoulders, legs, face, and forehead.

back, shoulders, and legs, while light touch on your face may relax your tightened jaw muscles, brought on by the stress of the day.

Older children five years and up have more body weight than a three-year-old does. I remember my daughter's footsteps on my back many a night after having a busy day at work. She would hold onto a wall so as not to fall off my back, or my husband would hold one of her hands as she walked from my neck down to my ankles and then up my back. On the folllowing page are some ideas for you to use when having your five-year-old massage your back.

WE ARE HERE TOGETHER

When Summer Raine, one year old, saw her sister Hailey walking on her dad's back, Summer Raine wanted to get in on the action. Guess what? With mom's help, holding her hand, Summer Raine took off and walked up her daddy's back, just as her sister had done, starting another family

ADDITIONAL ABC'S FOR DR. ELAINE'S TOUCHTIME MASSAGE FOR PARENTS BY OLDER CHILD (FIVE YEARS OLD)	
Ask permission	You may ask your child to give you a massage or your child may ask you if you want a massage.
Be involved	You and your child will mutually agree to the massage.
	You and your child will mutually respect one another, knowing that massage time is not a time to hurt anyone, but rather a time to make someone feel better, a time to show caring and tenderness, and a time of acceptance and acknowledgement.
Consider postures	You get to choose which position works best for you. You may lie down on the floor with your face down.
	Your child's weight on your buttocks can help your lower back release pressure and tension accumulated throughout the day.
	Your child may also massage your shoulders, legs, face, and forehead.
Select stroke movements	Your child may choose the types of strokes he wants to give.
	You can ask your child for certain strokes and with mutual dialogue determine the types of strokes you would like to receive.
	Your older child may walk up and down your back by alternating each foot starting from the buttocks, going up to your neck.
	Your older child's feet are parallel to your spine. (Do not have your child walk directly on your spine.)
	Your older child can also stand sideways with each foot perpendicular to your spine, moving up the spine with the weight in the toes and heel of the foot so the weight is only lightly on the spine.
	Your child can use percussive motions on your back like chopping vegetables. He can use gentle punching with an open hand or dabbing you with a cupped hand. This will be one time he can "hit you" without getting in trouble.

tradition. Using massage, families benefit as the family unit is strengthened. Each family member reads the cues of another. With mutual respect, closeness develops and caring is fully expressed.

I will never forget the picture I still see in my mind's eye of little Hailey, Summer Raine's older sister. Hailey had just finished being part of Dr. Elaine's TouchTime Baby Massage workshop at my Baby Steps clinic with her parents and sister. Hailey had told me, and even shown me, how much she loved to be massaged on her face. (See photo from "At Bedtime" on page 131.) Along with Hailey's family, Michelle, a family friend, came along to learn about infant massage. Michelle was seven months pregnant, extremely thoughtful and desirous of being the best mother she could possibly be for her newborn. She thought she would learn about infant massage so she would be prepared when her baby arrived. During the class, Michelle was given a doll to use to practice the stroke movements.

At the end of the workshop, I looked over to see the pregnant young woman sitting on a chair. Although she knew that she could sit on a chair during the infant massage instruction, she chose to sit on the floor with the rest of the folks learning about massage. Now she was sitting up on a chair and attempting to get more comfortable. As a child development instructor, I always tell my students to remember that children learn from models. If you want your children to behave in a certain way, then you, as role models, need to behave that way also.

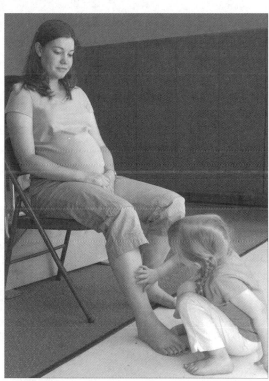

So while everyone was busy conversing and eating dessert and discussing their babies, I looked over to the side of the room where Michelle was sitting and saw a lovely sight—one that I preach about, but here it was manifested. Hailey, who was present during the workshop, who told me how much she enjoys receiving her own angels on her face, went over to Michelle, sat down on the floor by her feet and began massaging her legs. Michelle was delighted to be the recipient of her touch. When I asked Hailey what made her think of massaging Michelle's legs she said, "It feels good. I want her to feel good, too!"

My friend Karen just told me how, since her dad was diagnosed with blindness, they have become closer. She is able to sit with him and stroke his hand. He in turn is able to use his touch to connect with her. He is no longer able to see her cues, but he can feel them. By touching her shoulders, he knows how much tension his daughter has there as he offers her a shoulder massage. By feeling her back, he feels how much stress she holds there as he offers to rub her back. By touching her feet, he can tell how sore they are as he offers her a foot massage. The relationship she has with her father has never been closer than it is now.

How we treat our children is how they will treat us in return, and how they will treat their own children, in this circle of life.

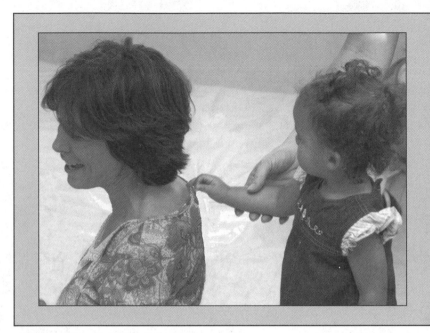

Dr. Elaine Gets a Massage, Too!

After I provided infant massage instruction to a group of parents, their babies, and the infants' older siblings, one of the toddlers walked over and started massaging my back. I was eternally grateful.

The pendulum swings from generation to generation. What we bring to our children will be brought to their children. How we treat our children will be how they will treat their own children. Massage is a lifelong process. We build bridges through our work and create more happiness, health, and relaxation as our voices touch and our hands speak. As much delight as we have from offering a massage is how much delight our children will have giving us the massage when all of us are older. Massage offers parents, grandparents, and other adults a way to bond with their children at any age, and in turn, offers their children a way to bond with their parents at any age, too. I can wholeheartedly say touch is ageless and transcends time.

CHAPTER 6

SPECIAL STROKES FOR SPECIAL FOLKS

The field of special needs is dear to my heart. Being a professional in the fields of early intervention, child development, psychology, communication, movement, and infant massage for over thirty-five years, I have seen the miraculous way touch heals and brings harmony to lives. I know first hand about being a child with a special need. As a child I was not able to clearly pronounce the "l" sound. The three words "I love you" that normally would mean so much when spoken to those you loved were like a dagger stabbing at my heart. Probably no one really heard the defect as much as I did. It wasn't until I was in college and received individual speech therapy at the Hunter College Speech and Hearing Clinic that I could finally say my maiden name Elaine Fogel accurately, and eventually corrected my articulation disorder.

What does this have to do with a book about baby massage? The important lesson is that when you are "hurting inside" or have a special need, the smallest difficulty is magnified and the ability of another person to touch you and connect with you means all the difference in the world. The following chapter shares with you ways massage has helped many infants, children, and families.

When I set out to write this chapter, I felt that I could best serve you to include areas we typically associate with special needs: attention deficit disorder, autism, cerebral palsy, Down syndrome, and spina bifida. And of course, no chapter on special conditions would be complete if not to include common gas, colic, and constipation. I also wanted to share with you other conditions of infancy and childhood, such as babies born via Cesarean section; with cleft palate or club feet; or in multiple births.

As society changes, we find that there are many different types of parents who are caring for children—grandparents, foster parents, adoptive parents, and day care providers—who sometimes spend more time with babies than the babies' parents. Babies being cared for by grandparents, foster or adoptive parents, or day care professionals often have their own kinds of special needs, too. In this chapter, you will learn facts about various medical conditions and some of the special folks for whom I have had the privilege of providing massage. You will see how to adapt strokes and how different interventions proved beneficial. Then you will enter the parents' world and discover how they learned about massage and the benefits it brought their child, their relationship, and their entire family. Children who are verbally capable of sharing their massage experiences will let you know what they felt. Some prominent healthcare professionals have also contributed their ideas and advice about massage and how it relates to everyone's well-being.

The National Institutes of Health is funding long-range research studies of the effects of touch on newborns, and has funded other studies using massage as alternative intervention for a variety of ages and disorders. Although we have a lot of work ahead of us, we are truly on the right path of exploration and discovery in learning about the benefits of massage for those with or without special needs, their families, and how this information can be assimilated into our everyday culture.

In the age of diagnosis, babies and children are given labels to describe their conditions. I prefer to label jars, not people. Nonetheless, in this chapter I have chosen to list categories of some special needs and conditions for your ease in reading. Please know that as a service provider and a governor appointee to the State of California's Early Start Program for Infants and Toddlers with Disabilities and Families, I firmly believe that children with special needs are *children first* and their *disability second*. You will see this reflected throughout this chapter when you read the following sections and read the label "a child with autism," rather than reading "an autistic child," or you read the label "a child with cleft palate," rather than reading "a cleft palate child."

GENERAL RULES OF THUMB

Your baby is unique, with a unique nervous system and unique experiences from which to grow. You bring uniqueness to every massage moment. However, the road ahead is often a bit bumpier a ride with a baby with special needs and conditions.

In this chapter, use the various Dr. Elaine's Rules of Thumb for each condition as the road map to take you to your destination. Use the various massage stroke movements as the streets that will get you there. You will aid your baby, give your baby calm and relief, and strengthen and tone muscles while growing your baby's brain. You will gain more confidence in your own parenting skills as you find ways to ease your baby's pain and discomfort. Your baby will thank you for it (if she can speak) and your relationship will improve.

Soothe, Strengthen, Securely Attach, and Smile

Using Dr. Elaine's TouchTime Baby Massage, you can accomplish the Four S's (soothe, strengthen, secure, and smile) with your baby or child with special needs and conditions. You will find a way to:

1. *Soothe* your baby:
So many babies with special needs and conditions are in pain and discomfort. By using Dr. Elaine's TouchTime Baby Massage, you will be able to offer her a way of easing her distress.

2. *Strengthen* your baby:
So many babies with special needs and conditions are in weakened states. By using Dr. Elaine's TouchTime Baby Massage, you will be able to strengthen her immune system along with other bodily systems, such as respiration, circulation, elimination, and respiration.

3. *Securely attach* and bond with your baby:
So many times you may be fearful that your baby's condition may worsen, you may hurt your baby who seems so fragile, or your baby may not be able to demonstrate affection. By using Dr. Elaine's TouchTime Baby Massage, you will become just a parent again, being able to recognize your child as a child first and connect with your baby at the primal level of communication, the level of touch.

4. *Smile* with your baby:
One of the most important aspects of life is to be able to smile and enjoy your time together, no matter how difficult the road may be. By using Dr. Elaine's TouchTime Baby Massage, you and your baby will create a time to laugh and enjoy one another through touch, by kissing each other on the nose, or in giggling while you move in harmony with your yoga stretches on your bicycle built for two.

Massage Strategies

Here are some overall massage strategies that I feel will be valuable for you. You'll find more specific information within each section on the various special needs and conditions faced by children and their parents and caregivers.

Dr. Elaine's TouchTime Rules of Thumb
Massage Strategies for Infants With
Special Needs and Special Conditions

- Always obtain medical clearance from your healthcare professional prior to beginning the massage to make sure that your baby's medical condition will not be compromised.

- Always check with other therapists who are seeing your child, if she is receiving therapy, to ensure that massage will not interfere with the treatment plan that they have designed especially for your child.

- Always individualize your stroke movements to accommodate your baby's unique needs, and your own. (For example, you may find yourself rubbing back to back as Caroline and Michael did, in the section on autism. You may find yourself stroking, with extra pressure, in circular movements on the lip area for a baby with a cleft lip as Tara and her son Brayden did, or Karen and her son Michael. Caroline also used deep pressure with her son Michael, who was diagnosed with autism, on his shoulders. Janine used brisk, quick movements with Patrick, who was diagnosed with spastic cerebral palsy.)

- Gradually introduce massage to your baby with special needs, since many babies with special needs or conditions may be insensitive or highly sensitive to touch. You may have to gradually introduce massage to them before they can experience the joy of touch with you. Cassady would flail her head backwards and try to squirm away at first whenever her mother would approach. After several days, a breakthrough occurred when Cassady stopped spreading her arms and relaxed under her mother's touch.

- Don't over-stimulate your baby. Massage is meant to be pleasurable, healing, calming, and even invigorating for those with special conditions. If stroking your baby is too stimulating, your baby will become disorganized, and unable to stay focused or relaxed. You may need to stop using that stroke, use another stroke, or adapt the stroke you were using. If there is too much sound (music playing in the background) adding extra sensory input to the massage moments, then take the music off. You can always go back to using it when your baby returns to a calmer state.

- Expand your idea of where and when you will massage your baby with special needs. Edgar's mother remembers the day Edgar was hurting so badly that he asked to have his legs massaged while standing up in the kitchen.

- Each time you massage your child, you will learn more and more about her. By massaging your baby, you can achieve dreams you may never have thought possible, and your child can come closer to reaching her full potential.

ATTENTION DEFICIT/HYPERACTIVITY DISORDER (ADD/ADHD)

Incidence:

- About 3 to 5 percent of the school-age population is affected by ADD/ADHD.

- Occurs in more boys than girls (although some say that not all girls are diagnosed).

- Chronic disorder that can begin in infancy.

- Diagnosed when a child is about six years of age and in a school environment.

- Exact cause of ADD/ADHD remains unknown.

- Neurologically based medical problem.

- Other research looks at diet and outside stressors.

- Some theorize that sensory deprivation or restriction of movement, during the period from infancy to about three years old, causes ADD/ADHD.

- An accurate diagnosis requires an assessment conducted by a well-trained professional—developmental pediatrician, child psychologist, pediatric neurologist, or child psychiatrist.

Characteristics:

Three specific areas of difficulty are attention span, impulse control, and hyperactivity (sometimes), with children requiring six out of nine criteria based on the standard Diagnostic and Statistical Manual of Mental Disorders. The criteria include: pays little attention to details; has short attention span; has difficulty organizing tasks; loses things; is easily distracted; fidgets and squirms in seat; has difficulty playing quietly; blurts out answers before questions are completed; and has difficulty awaiting turns.

Research:

Children diagnosed with ADD/ADHD and who were provided massage for ten consecutive school days showed improvement. The massage-therapy group rated themselves as happier and observers rated them as fidgeting less following the sessions. Teachers reported that the massaged students were more on task and gave them lower hyperactivity scores, based on classroom behavior after a two-week time period.

Dr. Elaine's TouchTime Rules of Thumb for Massage With Children With ADD/ADHD

- Check with your healthcare professional(s) to make sure there are no contraindications for massage and speak with any therapists who may be providing therapy to your child.

- Discuss the touch benefits with the child with ADHD.

- Get permission from your child with ADHD.

- Use moderate pressure and smooth strokes.

- Smooth strokes up and down the neck.

- Smooth strokes from the neck across the shoulders and back to the neck.

- Smooth strokes from the neck to the waist and back to the neck along the vertebral column.

- Apply calming effects of deep pressure, warmth, and stroking slowly and firmly down back for about three minutes.

- Apply deep pressure into the skin of the palm (in the inner space closest to the thumb between the base of the index finger and the thumb) for approximately ten seconds.

Daisy and Emily's Story

I am reminded of twelve-year-old Emily, who was accompanied to my clinic by her grandmother. Daisy was very concerned about her granddaughter, who was unable to concentrate and was having difficulty listening to directions in class and at home. Emily was fidgety and had many of the symptoms of a child with ADHD. Daisy wondered if there was anything she could do that would help her focus her granddaughter and learn how to calm her too. I spoke to Emily to gain insight about her knowledge of her difficulties. She knew she was having a difficult time focusing and wanted to improve herself. I spoke to Daisy and explained to her the benefits of touch and ways she could provide touch techniques with Emily to assist Emily's concentration. Both were agreeable to trying out the "touch techniques." I demonstrated how to use "joint compression" and smooth strokes on Emily's neck and back. Emily was agreeable in giving her grandmother, Daisy, permission to massage her. Several weeks later they returned to my clinic. Daisy was happy to tell me that Emily was calmer and the massage was helping Emily become relaxed and more focused. Emily also reported that she felt better after the massage and was happier knowing that she could have her body relax and make herself more alert and aware of her surroundings. Even Emily's teachers reported that they had seen a change in Emily in the classroom.

AUTISM SPECTRUM DISORDER

Incidence:

- Affects one in five hundred children.

- Occurs three to four times more in boys than girls.

- If a family has a child with autism, there is a 5 to 10 percent chance that another child will have the disorder.

- 0.1 to 0.2 percent chance that a child with autism spectrum disorder will be born to a family with no previous children with autism spectrum disorder.

Characteristics:

- Communication problems with spoken or unspoken words (verbal or non-verbal language).

- Difficulties in social interactions, whether through touch, hugging, or conversation.

- Prefer to be hugged on own terms, when they initiate it (according to Siegel, 1999).

- Obsessive with following patterns and schedules, "lining up" belongings, and repetitive behaviors (repeating words and/or actions over and over).

- Symptoms of autism usually measurable by certain screening tools by 18 months of age. Recent findings show that behavioral nuances and vulnerabilities are visible to the trained eye as early as 3–6 months of age.

- Parents say that at least 20 percent of children with autism experienced a "regression"—a loss of communication skills.

- Natural tendencies to "parent" (hug, kiss, comfort) are usually refused by child.

Research:

A study conducted by the Touch Research Institute in Miami, Florida, showed that children with autism who were massaged before bedtime, rather than merely read to, exhibited less stereotypic behavior and showed more on-task and social relatedness behavior during play observations at school. They also experienced fewer sleep problems at home.

Dr. Elaine's TouchTime Rules of Thumb for Massage With Children With Autism

- Check with your healthcare professional(s) to make sure there are no contraindications for massage and speak with any therapists who may be providing therapy to your child.

- Gain permission from your child, which will often be non-verbal.

- Don't expect any eye contact or a spoken "yes" to your question, "Do you want a massage?"

- Be an overly aware observer of your child's signs for when to engage. (See Caroline and Michael's story on page 157.)

- Be available to provide massage for your child.

- Accept one stroke (connection) at a time, building up to more strokes as your child tolerates them and subsequently enjoys them.

- See what body part your child likes having massaged and massage that part.

- Remove excessive stimulation from the environment if too over-stimulating.

- Follow your child's lead.

- Massage your child's shoulders, arms, hands, etc., with deep pressure, as tolerated.

- Enhances closeness with your child via an alternative method to verbal communication. (See additional benefits for parents in Appendix IV.)

Caroline and Michael's Story

Caroline takes us back to the time that her son Michael, now twelve, was thirty-six months old, and had just been diagnosed as autistic four months previously. Caroline says, "I was feeling confused, extremely sad, and determined to find something that would help my son." She found that the most disturbing thing to her was that her son didn't allow her to show any affection towards him. He was very often inconsolable and she felt in the beginning that he was her "alien" child. He tantrumed a lot and simple things like tucking him into bed at night and kissing him good night just "set him off" and caused him to scream, and scream, and scream.

Caroline attended a workshop I gave at a Governor's Conference for Early Start in California for infants and toddlers with disabilities and their families. On this day, I had invited parents and their infants to demonstrate and share massage. I also brought videotapes of many parents, infants, and young children engaging in massage and communication with their little ones. As Caroline watched several parents massaging their children, she thought, "I can do that!" She remembers me telling the audience to "accept what the child is offering you in terms of closeness and begin massaging when your child feels comfortable and willing."

Caroline began paying closer attention to her son's body language and one morning, she said, "It just happened. I was sitting down in the bathroom (you never know when the moment will occur) of my house in the early morning hours. It was a little dark and the house was quiet. Michael walked into the bathroom and backed up against me. I recognized his close moment and with his willingness, took the opportunity to massage his shoulders a little firmly. Almost immediately his posture relaxed. I continued for a few moments and then he walked away. I was so happy that he allowed this interchange. I started initiating more deep massages on the back of his body from his shoulders and down his back around his hips. He really liked it, and stayed with me longer. He began sitting on my lap or leaning on my lap. Then he started getting in my bed in the early morning and backing up against me for a massage. I felt like the Mama Bear and he was the Baby Bear. We had finally bonded with one another. He sought me out for comfort and allowed me to hold him and love him."

Michael is now twelve years old and is actually very affectionate. He still loves his back massages and deep pressure. Everyone who knows Michael comments on his affectionate personality and how he understands emotions in a real "emotional" way, unlike many other children with autism.

Caroline acknowledges how extremely important it was for her to bond with her child, and Dr. Elaine's TouchTime Massage provided an avenue for that to happen. In Caroline's words, "It was real; immediate; and brought us closer in a very fast and effective way. It was a technique that provided me with a skill greater than any other."

CEREBRAL PALSY

Incidence:

- About 764,000 children and adults in the United States manifest one or more symptoms of cerebral palsy.

- About 8,000 babies and infants are diagnosed each year.

- Each year 1,200 to 1,500 preschool-age children are recognized as having cerebral palsy.

- Faulty development of, or damage to, the brain's motor areas disrupts the brain's ability to control movement and posture.

- Early signs appear before eighteen months of age.

Characteristics:

Symptoms include difficulty with fine motor tasks (hands and fingers); difficulty maintaining balance or walking, or with motor skills; involuntary movements; frequent slowness in reaching developmental milestones, such as learning to roll over, sit, crawl, smile, or walk.

There are four types of cerebral palsy: ataxic, athetoid, spastic, and mixed forms.

Research:

Following one month of massage, spasticity and hypertonicity had decreased and perfomance on gross and fine motor assessments improved in children with cerebral palsy. Muscle flexibility improved along with positive social interaction.

Dr. Elaine's TouchTime Rules of Thumb for Massage With Children With Cerebral Palsy

- Check with your healthcare professional(s) to make sure there are no contraindications for massage and speak with any therapists who may be providing therapy to your child.

- Children who have cerebral palsy may have a combination of "high tone" and "low tone" working together in muscles.
  - A limp tone, like a jellyfish, may be referred to as *hypotonia*.
  - A rigid tone, like a stiff board, may be referred to as *hypertonia*.

- For infants with hypertonia (increased muscle tone):
  - Use slow rhythmical strokes down away from the heart.
  - On the back, stroke down in the direction of hair growth in a kind of swooping action.

- For infants with hypotonia (reduced muscle tone):
  - Use quicker, energizing strokes towards the heart.
  - Use more pressure as tolerable, but don't harm joints or tendons as in a rolling motion.

Janine and Patrick's Story

Patrick, two years old, was diagnosed with spastic cerebral palsy and hypertonia when I met him and his mother Janine, his brother Richard, and his sister. Patrick was in my Baby Steps early intervention program, receiving early intervention child development services in addition to speech therapy and occupational therapy. Patrick could not walk or talk. He could barely hold his head upright. He was carried by his mother or was pushed in a wheelchair to get around.

Janine followed the directions I had given her regarding massage for Patrick's stiffness. He was being "softened" and his muscles were loosening up as his mother used slow rhythmical strokes. Patrick especially enjoyed this massage before the other teachers and therapists came to work with him, because the massage gave him better range of motion, facilitated a sitting position with his head more upright, and enhanced his alertness for his other intervention. Dr. Elaine's TouchTime Baby Massage provided a special time for Patrick and his mother. Janine was able to make time to be together with Patrick and be present with her son. She did not think about what she was going to make for dinner, or who was on the telephone. As a matter of fact, she let the answering machine pick up any messages while she was massaging Patrick. The massage time gave them both a chance to relax and be together.

I will never forget the words that Janine shared with me about the benefits she felt that massage brought to her and her family. She said that before she learned how to provide massage with Patrick, he was "just Patrick" but now, since they started massage, Patrick had a personality. He had come alive for her and her family. Patrick, unable to communicate in words, was able to coo and babble back to her while she massaged his chest. She encouraged him and said, "tell me more." Patrick let the floodgates open and in a two-way communication babbled more than Janine ever thought possible. Patrick had a way with his sounds and it tickled his mother's heart as she lovingly smiled at her newfound son!

CESAREAN BIRTH

Incidence:

- Cesarean births deprive infants of physical touch.

- The National Center for Health Statistics found that in the United States in 2002, 26.1 percent of live births ended in C-sections. The rate of primary C-delivered babies was 18.0 per 100 live births.

- A baby may have to be born with a C-section for a variety of reasons: STD (sexually transmitted disease) may prevent a vaginal birth; breech delivery, whereby the baby is turned and her head will not readily move along the birth canal; prolonged dilation without producing contractions; or being in labor for excessive hours without the baby's head crowning.

Characteristics:

- Babies born through Cesarean exhibit biochemical differences.

- Babies born through Cesarean section may be prone to sluggishness, decreased reactivity, and less frequent crying than the vaginally delivered.

Research:

Results have confirmed differences between Cesarean and vaginally born infants. Cesarean babies desire more physical contact.

Dr. Elaine's TouchTime Rules of Thumb for Massage With Children Delivered via Cesarean Birth

- Check with your healthcare professional(s) to make sure there are no contraindications for massage and speak with any therapists who may be providing therapy to your child.

- Use your healing time as a way to get closer to your baby.

- Lie on your side and place your baby near you.

- Use holding, stroking, and caressing right now, while gradually introducing one stroke, such as stroking down your baby's back as she is held in your arms.

- Hold your baby, touch your baby, stroke your baby, keep her close to you.

- Simulate the womb, and offer your baby all the contact that was lost when she missed out on her monumental massage—her birth.

- Her closeness with you will also assist in stimulating contraction of your uterus, provided by the release of oxytocin (as mentioned in Chapter 1).

- Offer full body massage after the umbilical cord has fallen off or massage over clothing or without oil (as listed in the section for Newborn Strokes in Chapter 3).

- Remember the uniqueness of your baby and that it is necessary for you to read your baby's cues to determine which strokes to begin with and which new ones to introduce. (You may want to locate a local infant massage class in your neighborhood.)

- When you heal, you should be able to lift and carry your baby as close to your body as you can. In the meantime, massage your baby on the changing table, so she is at a higher level and you won't have to bend down.

Katie's Story

Katie was delighted that she was able to learn baby massage early on after her Cesarean. Although she was able to plan the exact day of birth with her physician and had everything straightened up in her house before going to the hospital, intuition said that her baby would need more touch than her other child needed. Although her baby's head looked just perfect after birth, and just about everyone told her so, she still felt that the important contractions never took place with this baby and she wanted to give her that experience, somehow. She figured that if vaginal births are nature's way of sending little ones into the world, than there must be a reason why. So now Katie is delighted that, by learning baby massage, she is giving her daughter the sensations of touch that were missing from her birth. She is seeing her daughter adjust to touch, and is happy with the health that they are both enjoying.

CLEFT LIP AND CLEFT PALATE

Incidence:

- Affects 1 out of every 700 newborns.
- Fourth most common birth defect in the United States.

Characteristics:

- Cleft lip: a separation of the two sides of the lip.
- Cleft palate: an opening in the roof of the mouth, in which the two sides of the palate did not come together.
- Unilateral cleft lip and/or cleft palate occur on one side.
- Bilateral cleft lip and/or cleft palate occur on both sides.

Research:

Massage works by kneading and stroking muscles to relax them, and stimulating soft tissues. This can increase blood and lymph circulation while breaking up scar tissue between muscle fibers. Although many of the families and professionals I have spoken with emphatically state that massage is needed to reduce tightening of muscles and keloid formation after surgery, there are no controlled research data with infants and children with cleft lips or cleft palates that demonstrate their beliefs.

Dr. Elaine's TouchTime Rules of Thumb for Massage With Children With Cleft Lip or Cleft Palate

- Check with your healthcare professional(s) to make sure there are no contraindications for massage and speak with any therapists who may be providing therapy to your child.

- Massage lips and mouth on the scars after surgery:
  - Rub in a circular motion on the lip area.
  - Use index finger or two fingers, depending on size of baby.
  - Use natural oil.

- Massage stomach using strokes for gas and/or colic symptoms. (See pages 174 to 175.)

- Babies with clefts may have air escape during feedings.

- Gaseousness and bloating may occur.

Karen's Story

Michael was born with an incomplete bilateral cleft lip. Karen reported that his cleft didn't go all the way up through his nostril. When his plastic surgeon, Dr. Stephanie Feldman, Assistant Clinical Professor of Surgery Department of Plastic Surgery, University of Southern California and staff plastic surgeon in the department of Plastic Surgery at Kaiser Permanente, Woodland Hills, saw Michael, she explained to Karen that his muscles seemed to be intact, but that the muscles in his lip were like a "tangled fish line." Dr. Feldman said she would have to go in and "pull everything down" to create a "normal lip and provide proper functioning."

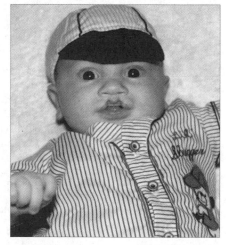

Michael at three months old.

Dr. Feldman believes in massage, especially after surgery. Karen reported that Dr. Feldman had asked her and her husband Paul to gently massage the "bumps" on each side of Michael's bilateral cleft "every time you can." Karen faithfully massaged her son's bumps before his surgery, and three weeks after his first surgery at four months of age, Karen massaged Michael's face and lips daily for thirteen months. She continued massaging his lips and the surgical lines for approximately four more years, approximately three times per week. These times were brief, and were faithfully done. Dr. Feldman told Karen what a great job she did massaging Michael's face and felt that the surgery was a success.

Karen also saw a lactation specialist to learn how to nurse a baby with a cleft. Karen recalls that Michael's lip seal was poor and a lot of air escaped while he tried to suck, which caused him great discomfort with gas and bloating.

Michael is a teenager now and there are no "knots" on his face. Although Karen reports how smooth his face and lips are now, future revision surgery will be warranted to enhance his facial appearance. Then it will be Michael who will be sure to follow Dr. Feldman's regime.

David, Michael's brother, reaped the rewards from Karen learning massage for Michael. Once David was born, Karen reports that she massaged both boys at bedtime, from their "heads down to their toes." Karen feels that the massage brought her and Michael closer together. It relaxed her and it was a special time for "mommy and baby." Karen said, "massage time was our time. Now as Michael and David are older, I still massage them and find it is a wonderful way to find out if anything is bothering them and stay part of their lives. Also, I get my own reward too because they now massage me back!"

Michael's Story

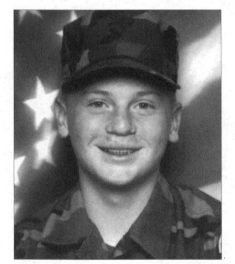

Michael at 15 years old.

Michael (aged 15) remembers that when he was a little "kid," his mom used to rub his lip, he would drink milk, and then he would fall asleep. "The massage comforted me so much," he said. "My lip had two bumps on it. It was cut into two parts. My mom would rub it and the bumps went down. It seems like a regular lip now instead of being all messed up. It barely looks like I have a scar anymore."

When I asked him about what he thought about massage, this is what he said: "It helped me out a lot. I healed faster. It makes it feel good. It relaxes you when you are a little kid. It makes you get closer to your mom. My mom and I have a really good relationship. I massage her and she massages me. She used to massage my feet, back, and stomach. I remember everything she did. I remember all of that."

In Chapter 1, I spoke about hormones and the brain. You can bet that so many pleasurable hormones were released during Michael's massage, and his memories are living proof of just how much we store this information throughout our body and remember them so vividly.

Dr. Stephanie Feldman's Comments
(Michael's Plastic Surgeon)

Dr. Stephanie Feldman said that parents should definitely try to touch their child so they see that the cleft is nothing more than something that can be corrected. Some cultures are afraid of the cleft, and so they don't touch the baby's lip. Other parents are just afraid of the cleft and don't touch it at all. Her advice after surgery is, "Massage, massage, massage. The more massage you do the better!" Since children are growing, when their lip is healing, they get thicker scars. The massage improves the scar, reducing the collagen build-up. Massaging the lip stimulates the blood supply into the area and softens the scar, which is good for healing.

The parent and child get in touch with what is there and they become an active part of the child's own therapy. Massaging the scar has psychological and physically healing properties. She further states, "I think that most plastic surgeons will tell you to massage a scar, although we don't necessarily look at that as massage therapy."

Dr. Feldman also recommends that you begin massage after the third week of surgery. (Also, check with your own healthcare provider to answer any questions you have about massaging your infant.) She said, "You usually get those 'bumps' (collagen build-up) about six to eight weeks after surgery. If you can massage a scar in this stage you can soften it. You can even massage it in the shower! Remember to caress and hold and massage those areas on your baby and don't be afraid. By massaging you gain better contact with your baby and develop better bonding as well as helping your child's physical healing."

CLUB FEET

Incidence:

- Affects 1 out of every 1,000 births.

- Congenital foot condition affects all the joints, tendons, and ligaments in the foot.

- Occurs more often in males than in females.

Characteristics:

- High arched foot.

- Heel is drawn up.

- Toes are pointed down, and bottom of the foot is pointed away from the body.

- The foot is twisted inward towards the other foot.

- The effected foot and leg may be smaller.

- The foot will lack motion and be noticeably stiff.

- The calf muscle may also be smaller.

- Commonly used surgical procedure for child of six months:
  - To release the Achilles tendon, it may be cut or released with a variety of procedures, to allow the foot to drop.

- Non-surgical treatment may begin when the child is three months old.

- There are frequent visits by a physical therapist who tapes and/or manipulates the foot.

Research:

There are no studies to describe the effectiveness of massage for children with club feet. I have had the fortune, however, of being briefed by many families about the benefits they've seen and will share a scenario with you in the section that follows Dr. Elaine's Rules of Thumb for Massage with Children with Club Feet.

Dr. Elaine's TouchTime Rules of Thumb for Massage With Children With Club Feet

- Check with your healthcare professional(s) to make sure that there are no contraindications for massage and speak with any therapists who may be providing therapy to your child.

- Straightening your baby's foot requires heel extension, which requires a stretchable and relaxed calf muscle, so:
  - Get permission from your baby for the massage.
  - Stroke downward on your baby's lower leg.
  - Hold the foot in one hand, and support your baby's calf with the other hand.
  - Hold your baby's foot and massage the calf.
  - Don't ever use force.

- Massage body parts other than your baby's feet to give your baby the greatest amount of relaxation.

- Allow your baby to re-experience her feet and freer movement after surgery.

Jennifer and Matthew's Story

When Matthew was born, Jennifer said, "I didn't know what happened. Now, I have so much information and knowledge that I am not scared like I was the first time I saw Matthew." Matthew was born with club feet. He had surgery at two months of age and got out of casting four months later.

He was then put into braces. The physicians cut his Achilles heel tendon, which was done in the doctor's office. Matthew has a few scars and his feet are often tender and sore, especially after medical surgeries.

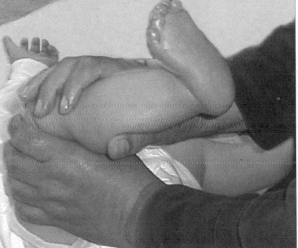

Jennifer said, "I find that I can massage Matthew's arms and legs, and other parts of his body that have not been invaded by surgical procedures." Jennifer has found massage to bring Matthew many physical and emotional benefits. The overall goal for Matthew is to be able to walk without braces. Mom said that after a massage, "I notice that his feet and ankle areas look straighter. His feet normally curve in and after they [are] massaged, I see his feet straighten out more. Even on myself, when I am massaged, I can feel the difference with my tension lessening. The massage relaxes Matthew and puts him to sleep."

Massage brings both parent and infant physical and emotional benefits.

Jennifer further said, "I see massage as a way of healing and relaxing Matthew, while getting close at the same time. My husband, Russ, is also able to massage Matthew and that brought them closer, too. I would urge any parent who has a baby born with club feet to bring them to a specialist as soon as possible. More children are born with this condition than you would ever know. You are not alone. It helps to get help early. Matthew is growing, and even trying to cruise furniture right now. I am happy to see his feet straighten more and more and know that massage is an answer for any parent who at first feels helpless, because massage is a way you can connect with your baby and he can connect with you."

CONSTIPATION

Incidence:

- 3 percent of all outpatient visits are attributed to constipation.

- 60 percent will have recurrent abdominal pain.

- Food, or not consuming enough liquid or roughage, may be the cause of constipation.

Characteristics:

- Stools become firmer and harder, and bowels are not emptied as often.

- Many times infants who are taking formula with iron, or those just beginning to eat solids, or both, may become constipated.

- Breastfed infants may digest more readily and have softer stools, and are less likely to become constipated.

- The hormone motilin also serves as an aid to increase bowel movement, therefore moving substances through the bowels. Babies who are breastfed have higher levels of this hormone.

- Intestinal bacteria can break down proteins more readily, too. Babies who are breastfed have more intestinal bacteria that can work at breaking down proteins.

- Your baby also may have colic pains, and be allergic to certain formulas, which can lead to constipation, or be introduced to solid foods when her digestive system cannot digest a certain food.

- Check with your healthcare professional if your baby is not gaining weight or shows other unusual symptoms.

Research:

In the area of constipation, I have not found any formal experimental research studies contrasting and comparing one type of intervention with another. However, there are innumerable anecdotal studies describing the vast improvement babies and parents experienced by using the various massage strokes that are listed below.

Dr. Elaine's TouchTime Rules of Thumb for Massage With Children With Constipation

- Check with your healthcare professional(s) to make sure there are no contraindications for massage. You may then use the following sequence of strokes:

- Daddy Longlegs; repeat three to four times. (See page 79 for this stroke.)

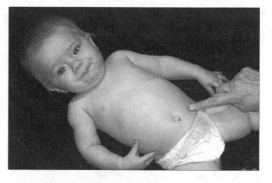

- Dear One (which is more of a smooth stroke with your fingertips starting at the 9:00 and moving across to the 3:00 and down in the shape of the number one); repeat approximately five to six times.

Stroking your fingertips across your baby's tummy in a clockwise direction and ending in the shape of a number one helps to move the fecal matter out.

- Earth Watch; repeat approximately five to six times. (See page 79 for this stroke.)

- Fanny Circles (on buttocks. These strokes may be done simultaneously or on one cheek at a time. They are also exceptionally powerful and can send babies going rather quickly, so be prepared).

  - Fanny Circles on right cheek: Take your index finger or your index and middle fingers on your right hand and massage the right buttock first, going clockwise about twenty-five times. Fingers should be only about one-finger width apart from the lowest part of the buttock separation.

  - Fanny Circles on left cheek: Using one or two fingers, circle counterclockwise on the baby's left buttock about twenty-five times.

Mom uses the Fanny Circles to reduce constipation by circling clockwise on baby's right buttock and circling counterclockwise on baby's left buttock.

- Fun Galore—Legs Up and In.
  - Hold legs bent into the tummy for twenty-five to thirty seconds.
  - Release legs.

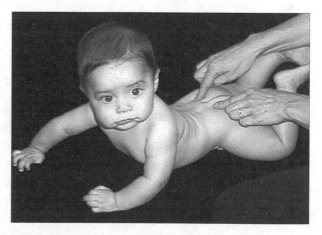

- Earth Watch; repeat five to six times. (See page 79 for this stroke.)

- Bicycle Built for Two; repeat five to six times. (See page 94 for this stroke.)

- Gentle Breezes. (See page 80 for this stroke.)

- Joyful Touch. (See page 75 for this stroke.)

- Repeat whole series three times, two to three times a day.

- You may also choose to shorten this series or adapt it accordingly to your baby's needs.

In the following story, Juana discovered one stroke, the Earth Watch, which resulted in assisting her daughter's bowel movement and getting her through her constipation. You, too, may find one stroke that seems to offer your child the most relief. Or you may find that a couple of strokes offer your child relief from constipation. The above set of strokes is not "written in stone." Observe your baby's cues to find the strokes that work best.

Juana, Anna, and Grandma Rosa's Story

Anna, thirty-one months old, had constipation, and the family physician recommended that fiber be added to her diet so that she would be able to have a bowel movement. At first, Juana, Anna's mother, reported that the fiber with plenty of water seemed to be doing the job. However, as time went by and Anna's body got used to taking that daily, her constipation seemed to reappear. Juana wondered what she could do to help her daughter, and Anna's grandmother Rosa wanted to help also. Both mom and grandma were instructed in Dr. Elaine's TouchTime Baby Massage for constipation.

Mom reported that, "The massage is just what Anna needed. She started having a bowel movement on a regular basis, going to the potty very easily, without any pain or discomfort. I found that a good time to massage her was after the bath because she was calm and she would give me permission. The one stroke I liked was the Earth Watch stroke. It seemed that one worked the best with her condition. My mother also could massage her and felt good about helping her granddaughter."

DOWN SYNDROME

Incidence:

- Affects 1 out of 800 births.

- Occurs in both genders, all races, and every economic group.

- Likelihood of having a baby with Down syndrome: Women under 35 years of age, 1 in 1,000; over 35 years, increases to 1 in 400; over 42 years, increases to 1 in 60; over 49 years, increases to 1 in 12.

- Although the likelihood of having a baby with Down syndrome increases with age, so many more younger women have children than older women that 75 percent of these babies are born to younger women.

- Cause is chromosomal disorder caused by an error in cell division.
  - Presence of an additional chromosome.
  - 92 percent of time Down syndrome caused by extra chromosome 21.
  - There are no known prevention methods.

Characteristics:

- Hearing loss (66 to 89 percent).
- Congenital heart disease (50 percent).
- Seizure disorders (5 to 13 percent).
- Cataracts (3 percent).
- Hypotonia—poor muscle tone.
- Hypertonia—possible tight muscle tone.
- Protruding tongue.
- Constipation.
- Spinal cord compression.
- Mild to moderate range of retardation.

Research:

A study from the Touch Research Institute found that children with Down syndrome had improved motor function and muscle tone following massage therapy. They had less hypotonicity, and they were able to perform better on fine and gross motor assessments.

Dr. Elaine's TouchTime Rules of Thumb for Massage With Children With Down Syndrome

- Check with your healthcare professional(s) to make sure there are no contraindications for massage and speak with any therapists who may be providing therapy to your child.
- Energize body limbs by massaging towards the heart.
- Reduce constipation by following constipation-reducing regime as described in the constipation section on page 169.

- Massage all body parts to energize movements and make body connections for body part identification and self-awareness.

- Massage muscles around the face area to assist with feeding.

- Move tongue backward into the oral cavity (massage inside the mouth to build greater awareness inside the mouth and make room for the tongue).

- Massage around the lips, starting in the center and moving out to the left and the right simultaneously.

- Use circular motions on the mandible joint, rotating the cheeks.

- Use massage inside the mouth on the roof of the mouth, with your finger making circles clockwise so that your baby can feel the inside of her mouth where the tongue is to stay.

- Close lips and ensure the backward movement of the tongue, making a smiling face on your baby's lips. (This can be done with toddlers and older children also.)

- Take your fingertips and place on your baby's cheek; stretch the cheek between your fingertips with one set of fingertips moving upwards and the other hand's fingertips moving downwards on an angle.

Mark and Ryder's Story

Dad and his son enjoy their time together as dad welcomes improved muscle tone and increased responsiveness.

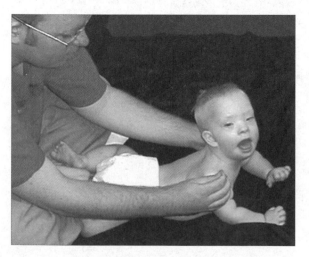

Ryder and his dad Mark were able to thoroughly enjoy the time they shared through massage. Mark especially enjoyed that he could see such a difference in such a short time. Ryder had hypotonicity in his legs. His dad was pleased to see the difference in muscle tone in Ryder's right leg after just a few invigorating long strokes. Mark continued massaging Ryder and then saw the different tone in his left leg too. Massage invigorated his muscles, and standing up became easier for Ryder. Mark let me know that shortly after he started massaging Ryder's legs, Ryder began walking. Mark attributes a lot of that to how effective massage was for improving Ryder's muscle tone. Ryder's responsiveness also increased with massage, and his lethargy reduced.

Mark and Ryder were always close, but using

massage, Mark discovered how much closer they could be. Ryder enjoyed their closeness too, smiling and laughing with his daddy. He loved his dad's touch so much that he never wanted him to stop at all, and mom saw how much fun they were having and wanted to learn how to massage Ryder, too.

GAS AND COLIC

Incidence:

- About 20 percent of babies get colic.

- Affects boys and girls equally.

- Cause may be related to digestive system, immature nervous system, or gastroesophageal reflux disease.

- Colicky babies usually have a healthy sucking reflex and a good appetite.

- Appears at about two to four weeks in breastfed or formula-fed babies.

Characteristics:

- Baby cries more than three hours every day for more than three days a week.

- Baby is usually healthy and well-fed, other than the uncontrollable crying.

- The condition worsens at night.

- Can last for three months or longer.

- Frustrating for parents, leading to high stress, anxiety, and difficulty coping.

- See your healthcare practitioner to make sure that your baby is not suffering from any other condition causing the fretful crying.

- Check different food ingestion and formulas to remove certain ingredients from diet.

Research:

Parents of babies with colic may feel helpless. Their relationship can suffer. Massage can alleviate some of their helplessness, as it helps them to be more proactive and they see that their baby can be soothed.

Dr. Elaine's TouchTime Rules of Thumb for Massage With Children With Gas and Colic

- Check with your healthcare professional(s) to make sure there are no contraindications for massage and speak with any therapists who may be providing therapy to your child.

- Use a full body massage to help your baby relax and fall asleep.

- Use the following colic stroke series to assist with removing gas from your baby's body and reducing colic symptoms:

- Dancing Half Moon; repeat three to five times.

  - As you face your baby, think of an imaginary clock on her tummy with her belly button being the center of the clock. Take the fingertips of your right hand and stroke from approximately the 9:00 to 12:00 to 3:00 on your baby's imaginary clock.

- Earth Watch; repeat five to six times. (See page 79.)

- Fun Galore–Legs Up and In.

  - Bring both of your baby's legs up into your baby's tummy while your baby is lying supine (on his back) or with you standing up holding your baby upright at your chest level while holding your baby's legs into her tummy.

  - Hold for about twenty-five to thirty seconds. (Watch out for the wind that can be passed while you do this.)

  - Release legs.

- Gently Kneading Kitten; repeat four to six times.

  - With this stroke, you might feel like you are a kitten kneading your fingertips on your baby's belly and allowing your fingertips to roll off your baby's tummy. Make sure you use both your right and left hands at the same rhythmical speed, assisting your baby's release of gas or relaxation from the pain.

- Fun Galore—Legs Up and In.

  - Bring both of your baby's legs up into your baby's tummy.

  - Hold for about twenty-five to thirty seconds. (Watch out for the wind that can be passed while you do this.)

  - Release legs.

- Gentle Breezes. (See pages 80.)

- Joyful Touch. (See pages 75.)

- Rub your baby's back to assist with calming and soothing, or your baby's head if that pleases your child.

- Repeat the entire sequence three times, two to three times a day.

- With a baby with colic, you may find yourself massaging through the crying. Continue to massage, using your best discretion. You may want to see a trained instructor of infant massage for guidance.

- Some babies respond well to the football hold. It looks like you are carrying a football; instead the football is your baby, and probably a crying baby at that. Place one arm under her torso by putting your hand through the space between your baby's legs. Your other hand can go under your baby's upper torso towards the shoulders. Move your baby on an even plane to the ground, like a glider. Your feet should be about shoulder-width apart and bend your knees. Keep your weight centered, as you may do this for fifteen or twenty minutes, just gliding your baby and soothing her with your movement. I remember showing Ben's day care provider, Jennifer, how to do that movement when he was just a couple of months old. She glided him in her arms as he cried until after about twenty minutes, he went from crying uncontrollably to complete silence as he fell asleep in her arms. (An extra benefit to Jennifer was that she felt she had gotten in some exercise for herself!)

- Another position for colic that you can try is one where you stand and hold your baby facing outward at your chest level with your baby's legs bent at the knees. This is a pose that Zohar tried with Sarah. Here is their story.

Zohar and Sarah's Story

At three weeks of age, Sarah had colic. She would cry from four or five o'clock in the afternoon to four or five o'clock in the morning every day. That's about ten to twelve hours all night long. This went on for three weeks. Zohar, mother and nurse practitioner, said she tried colic tablets, homeopathic tablets, gas drops, and headache medication. "Since I was breastfeeding Sarah," said Zohar, "I stayed away from all the foods you could think of, including broccoli and beans. In the end I lost forty pounds in three weeks and Sarah kept on crying." Even though Zohar is a nurse practitioner, she went to the doctor to make sure that her child

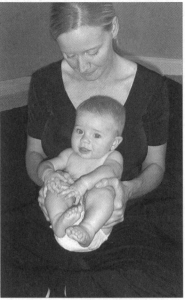

Mom holds baby facing outwards and with knees bent. If baby could talk she'd say, "My, what a relief it is!"

was okay, since she couldn't understand why her daughter kept crying so much.

Not everything was peachy keen. Zohar said that you must get somebody to help you—a spouse, relative, or friend. Zohar's mother stayed with Zohar and her family. "I cried," said Zohar. "I thought I was going to wring Sarah's neck. Then, fortunately for me, I was able to move to my parents' house. I fed her. I rocked her. I changed her. I needed somebody to help at nighttime or during the day to give me a break. I needed to know that I could walk away and put my baby down because she was crying anyway and I could get five minutes to get myself together. I felt rage, with my first child. You think you are doing everything right. You start off saying what a poor baby, then you say, poor me. If you can, get the help and know that you will get a breather, so you don't do anything that will make you upset or harm your own baby."

Zohar was willing to try anything to help Sarah stop crying. She heard about infant massage and then decided to see if that would have any effect on Sarah's crying. At first, Zohar explains, "Sarah didn't like infant massage. She cried and especially when I got to her tummy, she didn't like it at all. She would scream so much. You can easily give up and say 'Oh, she doesn't like it' and every time I started another body part she would cry." Zohar realized that she was not hurting Sarah and that it was just a lot of stimulation. "It took Sarah a while to get used to the strokes, but once she figured out that it was relaxing and she would feel good, then she wanted it.

"After approximately ten to fourteen days, she was a different child. She had stopped her crying. She enjoyed the massage and would look forward to the massage. When I got the pillow down that I always used with the massage, she would start to calm. My husband Derek was also able to massage Sarah which was great because this was a way that he could bond with her and they could be together.

"As far as I am concerned, infant massage saved me. It saved my sanity. It helped reduce Sarah's tummy pain and nothing I tried before would help. She still woke up, but she would have less pain. She could get some sleep and I could get sleep too."

Zohar massaged all of Sarah's body parts, but focused on her stomach. "I did the strokes like your Earth Watch and I sang to her and told her that 'Mommy loves you, and I am doing this to make you feel better.' I spoke in a calm voice. I massaged her legs with one hand under her leg and the other one on top of it. I used my thumb and pressed and rubbed the bottom of her feet and massaged and stretched her toes. This really didn't take too long, about five to ten minutes approximately. I remember rubbing her tummy with my two fingers, the index and the middle finger, following the path of her intestines and rubbing and saying 'Mommy loves you.' Then I wrapped my fingers and put them behind her back and some on the front of her chest and like hugging her I placed my thumbs on her stomach and rubbed up and down. I massaged her arms and hands, back and scalp. She liked getting the massage on her head too. Rubbing her scalp was like giving her a shampoo. Massage was the only thing that calmed down Sarah and changed her behavior."

Zohar said, "I have gained more empathy for other families and what they are going through. Before when parents of colicky infants used to see me at my work and share their story about their child being colicky, I would tell them, 'Don't worry! It's okay,' and walk away."

Now Zohar says she never walks away from any parent, especially a parent talking about colic. She knows what it is like to be in their shoes and she is better able to empathize with anyone who comes into her office.

MULTIPLE BIRTHS

Incidence:

- Less than 3 percent of all births are twins.

- Incidence of fraternal twins varies by ethnicity. (African descent: 1 birth per 70; Caucasian descent: 1 birth per 88; Japanese descent: 1 birth per 150; Chinese descent: 1 birth per 300.)

Characteristics:

- Even twins separated at birth will have many of the same idiosyncrasies.

- Identical twins exhibit almost identical brain wave patterns.

- Twins have a unique, intertwined life, being part of the same sac as identical twins, or sharing space within their mother's womb as a fraternal twin.

Dr. Elaine's TouchTime Rules of Thumb for Massage With Twins or Other Multiple Births

- Check with your healthcare professional(s) to make sure there are no contraindications for massage and speak with any therapists who may be providing therapy to your child.

- Be sensitive to the unique needs of each twin.

- Pay attention to their individual likes and dislikes.

- Feel their particular body structure and understand their unique emotional needs as well as their individual physical needs (one twin may be born with a shoulder or a neck that is strained from sharing space inside mom's womb or being at an awkward angle).

- Use the same strokes as listed in Chapter 3, adjusting your hand usage or finger usage depending on the size of your twin, and follow your baby's lead.

Katie, Gary, Sarah Jane, and John's Story

John and Sarah Jane are twins. I remember when John's dad, Gary, offered John his first chest massage. John began babbling and making sounds that his father had not heard before. When I questioned Gary about John's birth, I was told that John had a heart murmur. Now as Gary began massaging John's chest, John began "venting," speaking from his "heart" and letting his dad hear about his story. Gary just let John "talk and talk and

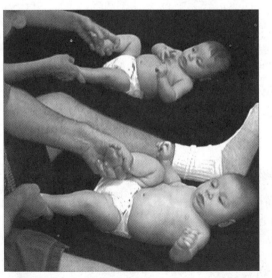

talk." He empathized with his son, and his son was safe and secure as he continued to communicate his story to his dad.

When Sarah Jane and John had their tummies massaged, and mom was massaging Sara Jane and dad was massaging John side by side, you could see the twins' harmony. Both brother and sister moved their legs rhythmically to their parents stroking as if riding a tandem bicycle. Synchronizing one's movements to the speech of the parent has been documented in science journals, however, in this massage moment the twins were synchronizing their own movements to one another with the rhythm of their parents' strokes. This was pointed out to Gary and mom Katie and it amazed them, since Gary had remarked that he didn't think John even knew Sara Jane existed.

The twins move in perfect synchrony on their own Bicycle Built for Two.

You may think a three month old may not notice his or her twin, but be assured that the touch and time they shared in their mother's womb facilitates their close connection, which unless we look closely, we may miss and not physically see or fully understand. (My mother and her twin sister had a remarkable understanding that spanned ninety years and went deeper than being a close friend. They often knew what each other was going to say before the other person said it!)

MULTIPLE CONDITIONS

Many of the children I work with have more than one special condition at a time, or multiple conditions. Brayden is one such sixteen month old who lives with his multiple conditions daily. His mother, Tara, and her husband, Joe, along with Brayden, are some of my all-time heroes.

Following are some descriptions of his conditions and the remarkable results massage has made in his short life.

Brayden's Multiple Conditions:

- Cleft palate. (See section on cleft lip and cleft palate, pages 162 to 165.)

- Gastrostomy tube: a device that is inserted surgically through the stomach wall, directly into the stomach. It remains there for a period of time and nourishment is put through the tube at designated intervals until the baby is able to swallow on his own without choking.

- Tracheotomy: an incision into the trachea (windpipe) that forms a temporary or permanent opening. The incision is usually vertical in children and runs from the second to the fourth tracheal ring.

Dr. Elaine's TouchTime Rules of Thumb for Massage With Children With Multiple Conditions

- Check with your healthcare professional(s) to make sure that there are no contraindications for massage and speak with any therapists who may be providing therapy to your child.

- Babies with multiple conditions are very fragile.

- Be flexible with no preconceived notion about how your baby will respond.

- It is always important to remember that the medical condition must always come first. If the timing is not right, remember that there will be other times for massage.

- Make a game out of the massage. Take one movement and make a funny face, or giggle, or kiss your baby's feet, etc.

- Let your baby touch your face, or put her finger into your mouth in her own exploration, and then you can mimic her movement.

- Always talk with your baby, and just like Zohar (page 177), let your baby know that you are not going to hurt her.

- Be prepared to focus on one body part at a time with your baby, until she begins enjoying the massage. When she does, you can then move on to other body parts.

- Babies with multiple conditions may not appreciate anyone going near their body to massage them. Many of these babies have had multiple hospitalizations with multiple surgeries, and multiple medical personnel poking, pricking, rolling, turning, and administering medicine and procedures all over them, especially on their faces (oxygen tubes), necks, (tracheotomies), and heels (blood drawn using heel pricks). These babies have every reason not to want anyone to touch them, and their muscles have the memories of those painful experiences.

Sometimes you just have to pick your battles. So if massage became too stressful for her child, mom would wait to massage him the next day. Nothing fixes overnight, yet the scars have become softer and blended into his face.

Tara and Brayden's Story

"Parenting a child with special needs is a high stressed job . . . I don't think anyone would ask for the job," said Tara, Brayden's mom. Brayden was born with an asymmetrical cleft with no palate and an open gap into his

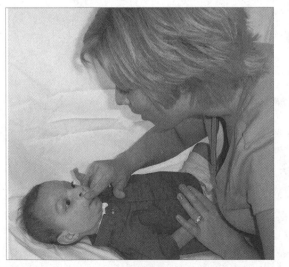

nostrils. He is sixteen months old now and has had ten surgeries. "When Brayden was born I was expecting a healthy, normal baby and went to every childcare parenting class I knew of to prepare for his birth. When I saw him, I saw the side of his head and saw something on his face and asked the doctor to clean off his face." Then the doctor flipped him over and looked at his face, took a breath and said, "Oh." Tara said it was as if her "soul had fallen out."

"It was the happiest and most mortifying time of my life," said Tara. She wondered what could have caused this to happen to her baby, and if anything else would be wrong and if she could have done anything to prevent it. Tara was devastated. Since Brayden had no palate, he wouldn't be able to breastfeed.

She had no bottles in her house and didn't have any formula either. She never thought she wouldn't breastfeed her baby. Now she had to learn a whole different set of parenting skills while feeling helpless and lost with her first baby.

At seven weeks old it went from bad to worse. Brayden had surgery after he had not gained adequate weight. Even though he was trying to suck from the bottle, he was burning up more calories than he was putting in. Surgery took place to insert a gastrostomy tube (g-tube) into his stomach wall. Tara could tube-feed him and build up his weight. Brayden had numerous other surgeries, and in one he actually suffered respiratory arrest, so a tracheotomy tube was inserted directly into his windpipe to make sure that he would get air. He also has had another surgery to resection his bowel.

Brayden had his lip repaired and had stomach surgery a couple months later. Tara discovered massage as a way of not only healing Brayden's physical scars, but also as a way to massage away emotional scars. She got her natural oil and massaged his scars almost immediately in a circular motion, and she saw the transformation and said his scar went from purple to pink and from pink to white. Tara said, "Brayden's scars were softer and looked better. I massaged his nostrils also. But I would play a game with him at first, because he didn't like me massaging his nose or lips." People looking or doing anything to his face traumatized him. Tara said, "I would play a game, like pinching his nose. Then I would apply a little more pressure, and he would throw up his hands as if to say, get away from my face! And if you put anything into his mouth, that was also a problem and he would throw a bigger fit."

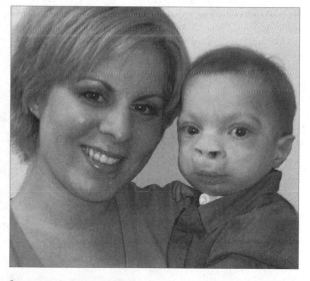

This mom and son are well connected and part of one big loving family.

So, she just put his hands on his own face, and then she would put his hands on her own face. Tara said, "We would just get together. I would massage him every day after bath time, whenever that time would be. I would massage his face every day and just made sure that no water would get into his ears since he had ventilation tubes. I kept lubricating and massaging his scars, and they were healing." She persevered and before long, she could see the improvement. It took Tara about one month until Brayden didn't fuss with the massage. As Tara said, "Sometimes you just have to pick your battles. So if he would seem to be too upset one day, I would try to massage him, but if it became too stressful, then I would wait to massage for the next day."

Tara continues, "My advice for parents is that nothing fixes itself overnight. Stick with it and you can do it for one minute once a day or two minutes or five minutes. Don't be discouraged if massage isn't working. At first your child may not like someone touching him. Make the environment as comfortable as possible. I always talk to Brayden and tell him, 'It's okay, I won't hurt you.' I always tell him what I am doing and I know that although he cannot talk back to me yet, he understands. Once he got the hang of it and knew I wouldn't hurt him, the massage provided great relaxation for Brayden and he is totally calm after his massage."

Dr. Janet Salomonson's Story (Brayden's Physician, Medical Director at St. John's Cleft Palate Team, Santa Monica, California)

I had the privilege of talking with Dr. Janet Salomonson about touch and massage at some length. She is totally supportive of massage and encourages physical contact between parents and children as a way for them to bond. She stated that, "Physically, scars do respond to pressure. Doing massage on the other areas could also help bonding and is great for the body to body contact."

Dr. Salomonson stated that she has seen scars heal faster than usual when being massaged, and that massage is a wonderful adjunct to healing. Her advice to parents who have children with clefts or multiple difficulties: "The child is like other children . . . he is a child with a cleft, not a cleft child. As a parent you try to relegate positive experiences that other children have and minimize the negative things."

Dr. Salomonson and the other team of physicians were so impressed with Tara and Brayden. She said, "Tara never lost sight of the first need and that was to be with her son. Whether in the pediatric ICU or at home, Tara provided hands on intervention and wasn't afraid of a tracheotomy tube or learning about sterile tabs. All of the physicians on the team were impressed with Tara and how she merged the technical with her intuitive mothering skills. Tara was successful interacting with her son, and not afraid of his medical condition that could have been frightening."

Tara and Brayden's respect and love for one another, interaction, and reciprocity are a tribute to them, and their relationship-based massage is a classic example of Dr. Elaine's TouchTime Baby Massage.

SPINA BIFIDA AND OTHER SPINAL CONDITIONS

Incidence:

* Affects 1 out of every 1,000 newborns.

Characteristics:

* Results from failure of the spine to close properly during the first month of pregnancy.

* In severe cases, spinal cord protrudes through the back.

* Surgery usually occurs within twenty-four hours after birth to minimize the risk of infection and to preserve the existing function in the spinal cord.

Research:

Dr. Robert A. Jacobs, head of the Division of General Pediatrics at Children's Hospital, Los Angeles, and his colleagues have stated in personal correspondences to me that there is not much research in the medical literature about massage and spina bifida. However, many anecdotes of improvement have been reported.

Remember that children with special needs are *children first* and their *disability second.*

Dr. Elaine's TouchTime Rules of Thumb for Massage With Children With Spina Bifida and Other Spinal Conditions

* Check with your healthcare professional and any other therapists working with your child to get a release to begin massage.

* Address your baby's needs, also remembering, as you would with any other baby, to make sure that you don't massage directly on the spine.

* Actively recognize your baby's developmental stages of growth.

* Bring awareness to, and stimulate, your baby's legs since sometimes there is partial sensation in them.

* Promote circulation. (By massaging you are keeping your baby's body in shape, so when your child starts walking or crawling she will have had good blood flow to that part of the body.)

Rose and Isac's Story

It is still difficult for Rose to speak at length about Isac's lumbosacral age-

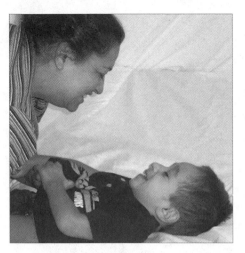

This little boy asks for a massage every night. Look how mom and her son enjoy their TouchTime massage.

nesis, a rare condition characterized by the absence of different segments of the lumbar spine, affecting bowel and bladder control. She is able, however, to talk at length about how much he loves his massage and how much she loves to be part of it. Rose says that Isac, aged twenty-four months, asks for a massage every night. It's a night time ritual. He can't go to bed without brushing his teeth and getting a massage on his legs. Rose said that Isac loves to pretend to be a pancake as she "flips" him over from his tummy to his back. Isac is very verbal and so Rose can ask him, "Do you want me to massage you harder?" "Do you want me to massage you more slowly?" "Where do you want me to massage you?" and Isac will tell her exactly what kind of stroke he wants, how he wants it, for how long, and exactly where.

Regarding physical conditions, Rose said that Isac's left foot would get cold and turn purple, but now that she massages his left foot the color is normal and so is its temperature. Also he used to have difficulty with runny stools. Since Rose has been massaging his stomach, the stool is more solid.

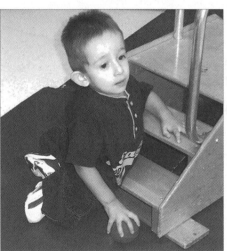

This little one is an inspiration. He propels himself around with his two arms, goes up and down stairs, and looks forward to being "flipped like a pancake" during his massage with his mom.

For a child who has such limited motor movement, Isac really gets around exceptionally well, and is truly amazing. He attends a karate class with his brother and loves to manipulate his body into so many different positions. He propels himself around with his two arms while his legs drag behind him. Massage continues to increase Isac's range of motion while enriching his relationship with his mother and Rose's relationship with him.

Desmond and Victoria's Story

Victoria is four years of age. She was born with spina bifida and hydrocephalus. She is using crutches to assist her in walking. Desmond is Victoria's dad and also a massage therapist. He has been massaging Victoria from about the third month after her first surgery. He sees massage as preventative. For example, he was told that his daughter was going to need surgery for hip displasia. She is four years old and has not needed that surgery yet.

When Victoria wears her crutches, her legs get tired. Desmond is able to massage Victoria's legs. Then she is able to put the crutches back on and walk some more. Victoria has learned a lot about her body and how to make her legs feel better. She is able to tell her dad, "My legs hurt" and request a massage with, "I'm ready for my massage now." Desmond massages her legs and helps to make her pain go away. Desmond feels that the massage allows Victoria to recover in half the time than other children in her condition.

Desmond sees massage as a relationship builder. He feels that massage has brought him and his daughter closer together. She can talk to him and share how she feels. Massage has also been a confidence booster for his daughter. She is able to tell her daddy when to massage her and she tells everyone how much she loves massage, too. She has a personality that is outgoing and exceptional.

Desmond's advice to other parents is that a child with spina bifida can do anything you allow them to do. Their hearts are bigger than anything. Don't hold them back. Let them know how much you love them. Desmond says that having Victoria has made him a better person.

GRANDPARENTS MASSAGING BABIES

I would be remiss if I didn't address these "special folks" who offer their own "special strokes." So many grandparents I have met want to give as much love as they can and find ways of being close to their grandchildren. The Touch Research Institute found when grandparents massaged children, their blood pressure lowered, they felt less depressed, and felt more willing to participate in life.

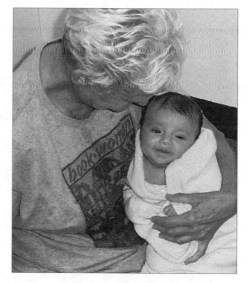

Sarah Jane and John's grandmother came to visit every Thursday. Her mission was to help her daughter who was blessed with not one baby, but two. Since grandma learned Dr. Elaine's TouchTime Baby Massage, she valued the time she came to be with her grandchildren even more. Now she found a definite way of bridging the generation gap and developing her relationship with her three-month-old twins by stroking, rubbing, and patting.

Grandma has formed a special bond with her granddaughter, providing her with ten fingers rather than ten toys.

Dr. Elaine's TouchTime Rules of Thumb for Massage for Grandparents

- Be in the moment. No one will wonder why you have wrinkly skin or gray hair, or no hair.

- Be in the moment when there is no parental interpretation about you or events that occurred with you and your own children, before your grandbaby's birth.

- Forge relationships, togetherness, and bonding with your own "touch signature."

- Enjoy your grandbaby being the center of your universe, feeling your love and being special.

- Transfer your knowledge to someone younger than yourself.

Linda and Melinda's Story

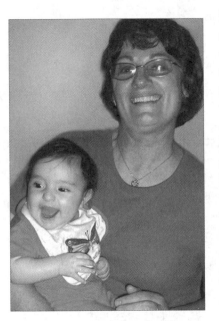

For Linda it was as if a light bulb went off. She had been concerned about how to get close to her baby granddaughter. She was wondering what she could buy her or get for her, and the answer was right there in her fingertips all the time. She didn't need any fancy toys or fancy CDs. All she needed to "plug in" were her ten little wrinkly, loving fingertips with her granddaughter, and for that matter that is all her granddaughter wanted, too. Through that human connection (which we are all wired for) of experiencing skin to skin, the youngest member of Linda's family would discover the true meaning of love, respect, and CARE. (See pages 18 to 19 for a reminder of CARE.)

Linda had the best time learning massage. She said that she never knew it would be so much fun. She especially enjoyed the time to ask permission from her granddaughter and learning how to observe her responses. Linda's daughter was also especially happy that her mother and her daughter could bond and develop such a loving way of getting close.

Happy grandma and grandbaby after their Dr. Elaine's TouchTime Baby Massage. "Oh we feel so happy, healthy, and relaxed!" This baby has discovered the true meaning of her grandmother's CARE.

FOSTER PARENTS AND ADOPTIVE PARENTS MASSAGING BABIES

Foster parents and adoptive parents open up their hearts and their homes to infants and toddlers whom they did not birth. Adoptive parents are full of love and giving. They have huge hearts to bring a child into their home. Baby massage assists these parents in bonding and finding their common rhythm. By learning how to massage your baby, you can learn about each other emotionally, and increase the physical health of your baby and yourself by releasing "feel good" hormones, while reducing stress hormones. (See Chapter 1 for more on this.)

Your new baby will be bringing information from another home, be that a physical home or a uterine home. Whether that home was of the biological parent or not, the rhythms and tone of your home will be different from the rhythms, tones, and aromas your baby was accustomed to in her old home. Sometimes the adopted child experiences much trauma because of her separation from her biological parent, so that the new parent may be pushed away. Studies show that 30 percent to 80 percent of children who enter into the foster care system do so with mental health problems, with 40 percent to 80 percent of these children experiencing some chronic health problems, 43 percent showing growth abnormalities, and 33 percent having untreated health problems.

When I taught a group of foster parents about massaging their babies, I was taken by the way these foster parents undertook their "mission" of bonding with the new baby in their care. They were eager to learn the cues of the newest member of their family. One foster mom reported that she saw how soothing and relaxing massage was with young children, so when faced with her 10-year-old foster daughter "going off" and "tantruming," she applied what she had learned and decidedly massaged her foster daughter's hand. Her daughter was generally out of control for fifty minutes. Now, after offering her daughter the hand rub, the foster mom said, "She was out of control for only ten minutes." This was an 80-percent change for the better. The foster mother was satisfied with her newly learned techniques and saw the universal value of massage for her new baby, as well as for her older foster child.

Dr. Elaine's TouchTime Rules of Thumb for Massage for Foster Parents and Adoptive Parents

- Check with your healthcare professional(s) to make sure there are no contraindications for massage, and speak with any therapists who may be providing therapy to your child.

- Don't take your baby's refusal for a massage personally.

- Allow your baby to grieve and "vent" about what has been lost and about the changes she has made or those she is facing. Left unheard, this could lead to destruction of any attachment and bonding that you may want to attain. Moving around from place to place and not being with biological parents, especially one's mother, leaves a void. The rhythms and signatures of the biological mother who carried this baby have deep-seated memories within the baby that transcend day to day events.

- Read your baby's cues. Go slowly with your baby. Trust will take time to build.

- Find your common rhythm.

- Massage through your baby's clothing, or start by holding a foot or a hand without stroking it, should your baby be hesitant about receiving massage.

- Gently introduce more strokes with different body parts as your baby accepts your touch (after massaging her legs for several days you can add massaging the feet).

- Slowly add additional stimulation, such as soft lullabies, songs, rhymes, etc. (See Chapter 4 for additional information.)

- Be patient in using your parentese voice to engage your baby.

- Follow your baby's lead. During baby massage you can learn about your baby, while allowing your baby the opportunity of leading the strokes, perhaps showing you the ones she likes. This is vital in the life of a foster or adoptive child who has been taken away from a biological parent's body, voice, and rhythms with which she had lived in utero. Now she has the chance to have someone listen to her as you follow her lead, and she becomes more powerful within your family unit.

Nancy and Jayson's Story

When Nancy was instructed in Dr. Elaine's TouchTime Baby Massage, she never dreamed that the massage would have so many benefits and bring her and Jayson, eight months old, closer than she thought they already were. Jayson had acid reflux. He was a "spitter" and a "vomitter" who had difficulty keeping food down. He expelled lots of gas. He had tight trapezius muscles and slept with a crooked neck.

   Nancy loved the idea that she would learn baby massage. She started massaging Jayson not only after his bath but also in his bath. In warm bath water, Nancy would massage his shoulders, tummy, and face. Nancy already felt close to Jayson, and felt as if he were her son even though she hadn't birthed him. She particularly enjoyed their massage time because she knew it was time for just the two of them to get closer, but also a time that was helping Jayson's body and bodily functions. Nancy reported that since Jayson has been receiving massage, his shoulders and trapezius muscles aren't as tight, his range of motion has improved, and he is sleeping differently. Before, he used to sleep with a crooked neck, and now his neck is no longer in that position. He also passed a lot of gas. Now he is moving his bowels better, spitting up a lot less, and his digestion has improved. Nancy finds Jayson much calmer now.

Nancy learned many stroke movements. She still knew that it wasn't the stroke itself that made a difference, but rather the relationship she was forming with her son that was most valuable. "I love getting home from work and having this cuddly, loving time for him and me," said Nancy. "Giving Jayson a massage helps me unwind from my day too. It is so positive because it brings such a fast connection with your child. He is cuddlier. He likes the sensory feeling. He loves the water so much and after the bath he loves the massage. He used to cry so much when you tried to move his arms upward. He would be fighting the therapist. But now he is happy when you move his arm and has no more resistance."

Nancy said for her and Jayson, "the massage provides a connection, touching, feeling, conversation, facial expressions, bonding, calming, [which are] very necessary in today's world."

THE "SURROGATE PARENTS" AT YOUR DAY CARE CENTER

What happens when you say good-bye to your little one at the door of the day care center? Do you ever wonder how your touch will be missing from your baby's day? Do you wonder how your baby is getting along without you? As I have presented infant massage around the country, I have been able to provide training for day care providers who have the task of being a "surrogate parent" while biological or adoptive parents attend to their daily activities. I say surrogate parents because sometimes so many of these little ones spend more of their waking day with their day care providers than they spend with their own parents.

What is exciting, however, is that once the day care providers have obtained permission from parents to massage their babies, they can help the babies relax and calm themselves to sleep at nap time or during the day. I am reminded of Ann, a day care provider at a day care center, who told me that after learning massage and obtaining permission from the parents of children in her charge, she found it so much easier to help the children take naps. By using long easy strokes on the children's backs and legs, she was often able to relax them into deeper sleep at nap time. She also found herself feeling more in touch with the children as her bonds with each one deepened. She was able to know more about each infant and toddler, and enjoyed understanding them more. The children also came to understand that there was someone in the room who cared about them and whom they could turn to when they needed comfort or attention.

Research from the Touch Research Institute supports what Ann noticed. Field and others found that preschool children who received massage fell asleep sooner and slept longer during nap time, and had decreased activity levels and better behavior ratings. Also, preschoolers who received fifteen minutes of massage a day were more alert, more responsive, and able to sleep more deeply. They also showed better performance with their thinking skills as measured by their performance on the block design and the pegs subsets of the WPPSI, a test that measures cognitive abilities.

Dr. Elaine's TouchTime Rules of Thumb for Massage for Day Care Providers

- Always get permission from the parent to provide massage for a baby or child in your care.

- Provide information about the benefits of massage to the parents in written literature, if possible, in the parent's primary language to promote full understanding.

- Always ask the child's permission to provide a massage.

- Read the child's cues and learn when the child might be more receptive to a massage, or stroking (before she lies down for a nap, or as a way to facilitate waking up from a nap). You might make a note of what times the child becomes fussy and offer a massage, with the child's permission, before that fussy time.

- Follow the child's lead.

- With infants or toddlers who are not potty trained, you may find that you may get their permission for a massage during diaper changing time, as you gently talk with the child. Keeping a bottle of natural oil close to the diaper changing table may facilitate massage of the legs, arms, or tummy.

- Let the parent know how the baby enjoyed the massage or if she did not.

- Encourage the parent to provide massage with baby at home, as a way of bonding, relating, and having some together time after a long day apart.

- Remember that even though you may be the surrogate parents for ten or possibly fourteen hours a day, you are not the parent and must respect parental wishes and desires.

- Respect different cultural backgrounds of your families who may have different preferences of being touched or massaged.

- Allow for individual differences within each culture.

Anna and Anthony's Story

Anthony had difficulty calming down at nap time. All of the other children were able to eat their lunch, have a "potty break," and go to their blue cots to lie down. Anthony would be walking around the room with his blankie in hand meandering from corner to corner and crying as the other children easily drifted off to slumber-land. Anthony was unable to settle down on the cot, and Anna didn't know what she could do. She tried to console him. She tried to talk to him. She read him a book. Nothing seemed to work until she obtained permission from his mother to try massage.

Before all the children were getting ready for nap time, she brought Anthony closer to her and held him. Then, with his permission, she would massage his back. She would move toward his cot and sit with him, massaging his back and legs right through his clothing. This took several days, and then Anthony began to relax right under her fingertips. "I was always so worried about Anthony. I didn't know what I could do to help him. When I learned about massage I found a way of helping him and myself. He is calmer now. The room is quieter at nap time, too."

I have worked with so many children with special needs and their families over my thirty-five years in the field of child development. I am grateful for the many parents who agreed to share their stories with you, so you could see how vital touch is in their lives, and the strength that massage has given them in getting to know their child *first* and their disability *second*. These parents are certainly the heroes and warriors in everyday life. Now, should you have an infant or child with special needs, you will have a foundation upon which you can build your very own relationships and become warriors too. These stories are only a few of the hundreds and thousands yet to be told.

As I end this chapter, I leave you with the following poem:

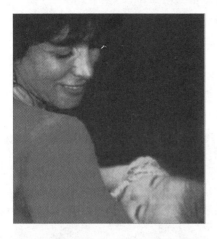

The Miracle Is You
—Elaine Fogel Schneider 2005

Don't be afraid
To smile amidst the tears
For you are a sensitive soul
Getting stronger through the years

Your baby came into this world
With you as her shield
As strong as your baby is to have survived
Don't ever think you've failed.

Never stopping for a minute
Always reaching for the stars
You touch the miracle of life
As you stroke your baby's loving arms

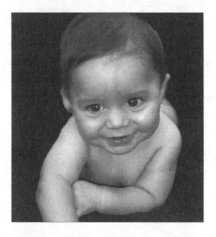

Watching and wondering
You find enjoyment too
For you are the warrior
The miracle is you.

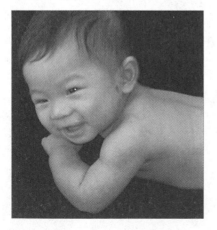

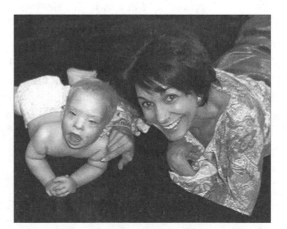

CONCLUSION

Thank you for joining me on this exciting journey. At no time before in history have we had the advantage of science showing us the valuable benefits and importance of touch, and the destruction of human survival without it! At no other time in history has the importance of relationships been so vital so that our children grow and learn about respect, compassion, and tolerance. At no time in history has it been so critical that we lay the foundation of trust and security for our infant than it is now. Never before have we had the opportunity of exploring the mind, body, and spirit connection as we do now!

You have seen how massage creates a dialogue between two willing individuals and how this relationship shapes the development of the brain's function and structure. You have seen how massage reduces stress by releasing or reducing hormones, strengthening immune systems, and growing both sides of the brain. You have seen how babies' sense of touch is awakened in utero, how babies are "wired" prior to birth, and how environmental influences affect the "use it or lose it" pruning of baby's neurons. By now you also realize just how vital the first three years of life are to your baby, and how significant the sense of touch is in your baby's development, health, happiness, and overall well-being—and yours, too.

In this technological world we live in, the vital sense of touch can easily be forgotten. You can put your baby in a carrier, in a carriage, in a crib, or in a swing, and the elements of touch can be missing from your everyday encounter with your baby. Now that you have learned so much about touch and Dr. Elaine's TouchTime Baby Massage, you shall be able to nurture your baby's growth through the magic of your own fingertips and the relationship you build together. Whether you have the time to offer your baby a full massage or only time for an abbreviated one, through massage your two bodies blend as one. Through the rhythms of your own breath and energy, you harmonize with one another. Whether using spoken words that resonate through your ears, or using unspoken words that resonate in your hearts, massage offers you and your baby magical moments that will resonate for a lifetime.

By integrating massage and touch into your daily life with your baby, you will be giving your baby a gift of a secure attachment right from the beginning of your relationship, fostering your baby's health, happiness, and serenity. This is a marvelous time on your baby's path of discovery in learning more about himself and the world in which he was born.

All parents yearn to be able to have lasting relationships with their children that will endure over time. Integrating baby massage into your daily life will allow you to create this path to your future. Dr. Elaine's TouchTime Baby Massage:

- allows your baby to learn about himself and his relationship with others;

- lowers stress hormones, which improves your baby's immune system, which leads to greater overall health and well-being;

- helps your baby feel a sense of control and predictability while loving rituals are developed;

- creates a special time for your baby so he will feel noticed and receive attention by being touched in a compassionate, gentle, and loving way (like how when Jacob saw his mother massaging his sister, Cassady, he wanted some special time with mom, too);

- allows you the opportunity to engage physically and emotionally with your baby, stroking him, talking to him, comforting him, enjoying each other while "structuring" his brain;

- allows you the opportunity to listen to your baby and respond to your baby while celebrating your baby's uniqueness, which furthers your baby's feelings of being worthy and loved;

- allows you the opportunity to read your baby's body language while you respond sensitively to his needs, building a safe and secure attachment, which promotes neural synchrony in your baby's brain, according to Daniel J. Siegel, author of *The Developing Mind*. When babies have secure attachments, they are ready to learn and are happier;

- allows you to learn about yourself and your relationship with your baby;

- lowers your own stress hormones and blood pressure level, so that you are more relaxed, which leads to your own greater overall health and well-being;

- need not be just for your "babies."

If you have picked up this book and have older children, it is still not too late to relate. As you massage your little one, your older child may be watching, and if he is like Jacob, he will want his own massage moments from you, too.

By reading your baby's cues and following your baby's lead, you are showing your baby or child that you understand when he wants a massage and when he does not. You are showing him that you understand what parts of his body he enjoys having massaged, and which ones he does not, and what rhythm, pressure, and flow he enjoys in the effort/shape of your touch. This translates into his feeling important. He sees your responsiveness to his needs, and that he matters in this world. When you are willing to see the world through your child's eyes, you are attuning with him and this helps build his security and balances his body, emotions, and states of mind. This is true love.

Through massage, as your child grows into an adult, he will have experienced that you will always be there for him. Your child will know that you have a special place in your heart only for him and he will be able to count on you forever.

By giving your baby a massage after bath time every night, or during the day at a specific time, you are developing a habit. By swishing your hands together with oil prior to his massage and asking permission ("Do you want a massage?"), you are helping him establish routines to transition from one state of awareness to another. In a world that is forever changing, routines and rituals build confidence and bring people closer. Being a confident child will lead your child to becoming a confident, flexible, and resilient adult.

When your baby starts fussing and disengaging during the massage and you stop for a cuddle break, kiss, or hug, you are demonstrating your affection for your baby. This tells your baby that he can count on you to read his cues and that you will always be unselfishly there for him. He is not alone.

When you are massaging your baby you are both having fun! Reciting rhymes or singing songs while massaging ("Round and round we go with your little toe" or "Darling baby you're so sweet, from your arms down to your feet") brings out the giggles. You can also have fun doing your yoga harmony exercises after massage. Your baby becomes comfortable within his own body and gains respect for the magnificent "temple" that he inhabits daily. He will know where his boundary ends and where other bodies begin. He will be able to competently take charge of himself, and fully express his needs physically, mentally, and spiritually.

According to Robert Noah Calvert, founder of *Massage Magazine*, the Western world is the last frontier for infant massage. By massaging your baby, and learning these effective techniques, you have the opportunity of starting family traditions and rituals, which will be pleasurably remembered by your child for years to come. You have at your fingertips the ability to build the foundation for a lifelong respectful and trusting relationship between your baby and you—one filled with happiness, health, and peacefulness.

Everyone has a message within us waiting to get out. I am not alone in my love for poetry and the desire to share with you the many verses I have written about massaging your baby. Years ago, while learning the art of infant massage, I wrote my first poem about the gift of life and the sense of touch and massage. So moved was I by the miracle of baby massage, discovering the child within me, the essence of communication through touch, caring, and genuine love for another human being that my poem, *A Joyous Welcome*, was penned. The words came to me while sitting at the edge of the Seal Rock Bay in northern California, listening to the waves ebbing and flowing upon the shoreline after completing one day of infant massage training. May your days be filled with beautiful massage moments. From my heart to your hands . . .

A Joyous Welcome

© Elaine Fogel Schneider, PhD, 10/20/94

Through the power of massage,
I accept you for who you are.
Through the power of massage
I acknowledge all I have to give.
Listening, watching and touching
The first language of our hearts
Beats a joyous welcome,
For you are a gift and
You are the memories I want to share.
With a firm and gentle touch
I say, "I'm here!"
I respect you,
I'll cherish you, nurture you,
Comfort you and protect you.
I'll laugh with you, cry with you
And drying away your tears,
Most of all,
With a firm and gentle touch
I say, "I'm here!" and
I will love you forever.

ℛEFERENCES

Chapter One

Ackerman, D. (1990). *A Natural History of the Senses.* New York: Vintage Books.

Acredolo, L., and Goodwyn, S. (2000). *Baby Minds.* New York: Bantam Books.

Ainsworth, M. (1979). Infant-mother attachment. *American Psychologist,* 34 932–937.

Ainsworth, M. (1974). Infant-mother attachment and social development. In M. Richards, (ed.) *The Introduction of the Child into a Social World.* London: University Press, 99–135.

Barnard, K. (1996). *Beginning Rhythms.* Seattle, WA: NCAST Publications.

Barnard, K., and Brazelton, T. (eds) (1990) *Touch: The Foundation of Experience.* Madison: Connecticut: International Universities Press, Inc.

Begley, Sharon. (1997, Spring/Summer). How to build a baby's brain. *Newsweek* Special Issue., 28–32.

Bowlby, J. (1969). *Attachment and Loss* (Vol. 1). London: Hogarth Press.

Bowlby, J. (1989). *Secure and insecure attachment.* New York: Basic Books.

Brazelton, T.B. *Maternal Attachments and Mothering Disorders.* Symposium by Johnson and Johnson, October 18–19, 1974, p. 54.

Brazelton, T.B., and Cramer, B. (1990). *The Earliest Relationship.* Reading, Massachusetts: Addison-Wesley.

Brazelton, T.B., and Greenspan, S. (2000, Fall/Winter). Our window to the future. *Newsweek* Special Issue, 34–36.

Calvert, R. (2002). *The History of Massage.* Rochester, Vermont: Healing Arts Press.

Condon, W. and Sander, L. (1974/June). Neonate movement is synchronized with adult speech. Interactional participation and language acquisition. *Science,* 183.

Cooper, G., Hoffman, K, Marvin, R., and Powell, B. (2000) Circle of Security Intervention Project. Spokane, WA, and Charlottesville, Va. www.circlesofsecurity

Cultivating the Mind. (1997, Spring/Summer). *Newsweek* Special Issue, 38–39.

Davis, Phyllis.(1999). *The Power of Touch.* Carlsbad; California, Hay House.

Diamond, M. and Hopson, J. (1998). *Magic Trees of the Mind.* New York: Penguin.

Eliot, L. (2000). *What's Going On In There? How the Brain and Mind Develop in the First Five Years of Life.* New York: Bantam.

Field, T. (1990) *Infancy. The Developing Child.* Cambridge, Mass.: Harvard University Press.

Field, T. (2001). *Touch.* Cambridge, Mass.: MIT.

Field, T. (1995). *Touch in Early Development.* Mahwah: New Jersey: Lawrence Erlbaum Associates.

Goldstein, SF. Massage helps develop a regular sleep cycle. (2002). *Journal of Developmental and Behavioral Pediatrics.* 23:410–415.

Gopnick, A., Meltzoff, A., and Kuhl, P. (1999). *The Scientist in the Crib.* New York: William Morrow and Company.

Greenspan, S. (1999). *Building Healthy Minds.* New York: DeCapo Books.

Greenspan, S. (2002). *The Secure Child.* Cambridge, Mass.: DeCapo Press.

Gunnar, M. (1996). *Quality of care and the buffering of stress physiology: Its potential in protecting the developing human brain.* University of Minnesota Institute of Child Development.

Gunzenhauser, N., (ed.) (1989). *Advances in Touch.* Florida: Johnson and Johnson.

Harlow, H. "Love in Infant Monkeys," *Scientific American,* 200:68–74, June, 1959.

Hart, B. and Risley, T. (1995). *Meaningful Differences in Everyday Experiences of Young American Children.* Baltimore, MD: Paul H. Brookes

Hawley, T. (1998). "Starting Smart: How Experiences affect brain development. An Ounce of Prevention Fund and Zero to Three Paper." Chicago: Illinois

Healy, J. (2004). *Your Child's Growing Mind.* New York: Broadway Books.

http://beta/communinty servers.com

Heller, Sharon. (1997). *The Vital Touch.* New York: Holt.

Izard, C., Porges, S. Simon, R. Haynes, O., Hyde, C., Paris, M., and Cohen, B. (1991). Infant cardiac activity: Developmental changes and relations with attachment. *Developmental Psychology.* 27: 432–439.

Kelly, J. and Barnard. (2000). Assessment of parent-child interaction: Implications for early intervention. In Shonkoff, J and Meisels, S. (eds). *Handbook of Early Intervention.* New York: Cambridge University Press. 258–288.

Klaus, M., Kennell, J., and Klaus, P. (1995). *Bonding: Building the foundations of secure attachment and independence.* Reading, Mass.: Addison Wesley.

Klaus, M., and Klaus, P. (1998). *Your Amazing Newborn.* Reading, Mass.: A Merloyd Lawrence Book.

Klaus, M., and Kennell, J. Maternal Attachment: Importance of the First Post-Partum Days," *The New England Journal of Medicine,* 286:460–463, March 2, 1972.

Klaus, M., and Kennell, J. (1982). *Parent-Infant Bonding.* St. Louis, Missouri: C.V. Mosby.

Kotulak, R. (1996). *Inside the Brain.* Kansas City: Andrews and McMeel.

Lally, J. (1997). "Brain development in infancy: A critical period." *Bridges* 3:1 Sacramento, CA: California Department of Education, 4–6.

LeBoyer, Frederick. (1976). *Loving Hands.* New York: Knopf.

Mead, M., and Macgrefor, F. (1952). *Growth and Culture.* New York: G.P. Putnam's Sons. 42–43.

Mead, M., and Newton, N. (1967). Cultural patterning of perinatal behavior. *Childrearing: Its social and psychological aspects.* Baltimore: Williams and Wilkins.

Melzack, R. and Wall, P. (1988). *The Challenge of Pain.* London: Penguin.

McClure, V. (2000). *Infant Massage: A Handbook for Loving Parents.* New York: Bantam.

Montague, A. (1986). *Touching: The Human Significance of the Skin.* New York: Harper and Row.

National Research Council and Institute of Medicine. (2000). Nurturing relationships. In J.P. Shonkoff and D.A. Philips, (eds). *From Neurons to Neighborhoods.* Committee on Integrating the Science of Early Childhood Development. Washington, D.C.: National Academy Press, 225–266.

Pawl, J. (1995/February/March). The therapeutic relationship and human connectedness: Being held in another's mind. *Zero to Three,* 1–5.

Pearce, JC. (2004, Spring). "The Conflict of Interest Between Biological & Cultural Imperatives. A survey of technological birth & its impact." *Touch the Future.* 8–12.

Perry, B. (2003, May). "The power of early intervention: The impact of abuse and neglect on the developing child." Paper presented at Los Angeles County Department of Mental Health Infant-Early Childhood & Family Mental Health Services Program (IECFMHSP) Initiative, Los Angeles, CA.

Pert, CB. (1997). *Molecules of Emotion.* New York: Scribner.

Peyser, M., and Underwood, A. (1997, Spring/Summer). "Shyness, sadness, curiousity, Joy. Is it nature or nurture?" *Newsweek* Special Issue. 60–63.

Porges, S. (1976). "Peripheral and neurochemical parallels of psychopathology: A psycho-physiological model relating autonomic imbalance to hyperactivity, psychopathy, and autism." *Advances in Child Development and Behavior*, 11, 33–65.

Porges, S. and Fox, N. (1986). "Developmental Psychophysiology." In M. Coles, E. Donchin, & S. W. Porges, (eds.) *Psychophysiology*. New York: Guilford Press.

Ramey, C., and Ramey, S. (1999). *Right from Birth*. New York: Goddard Press.

Ranpura, A. A Conversation with Marian Diamond. www.brainconnection.com (2004, April 4).

Raymond, J. (2000, Fall/Winter). "The world of the senses." *Newsweek* Special Edition, 16–18.

Schneider, EF. (2001, May). "Therapeutic infant massage." Paper presented to Cedars Sinai Mental Health Initiative First Five. Los Angeles, CA.

Schneider, EF. (1996, January). "The power of touch. Massage for infants." *Infants and Young Children*. 8(3), 40–55.

Schneider, EF. (1997, July/August). "Touch communication: The power of infant Massage." *Massage Magazine*, 40–43.

Schneider, EF. (2002, March). "Recent Research and Relationship-Based Early Intervention Communication." Paper presented at the meeting of a collaboration Between the Infant Development Association of California and the California Speech-Language-Hearing Association. Los Angeles, CA.

Schore, A. (1994). *Affect Regulation and the Origin of the Self*. Hillsdale, New Jersey: Lawrence Erlbaum.

Shore, R. (1997). *Rethinking the Brain*. New York: Families and Work Institute.

Siegel, D. (1999). *The Developing Mind*. New York: Guilford

Siegel, DJ. (2004, December). "Attachment and Self-Understanding: Parenting with the Brain in Mind." Paper presented at the 0–3 Conference, Sacramento, CA.

Siegel, DJ. "Toward an Interpersonal Neurobiology of the Devleoping Mind: Attachment Relationships, "Mindsight," and Neural Integration." *Infant Mental Health Journal*. 22(1–2), (2001); 67–94.

Stein, R. (2004, Spring). "Disease tendencies begin in womb." *Touch the Future*. 5–7.

Stern, Daniel.(1998). *Diary of a Baby*. New York: Basic Books.

Stroufe, A., Egeland, B., Kreutzer, T. (1990). "The fate of early experience following developmental change: longitudinal approaches to individual adaptation in childhood." *Child Development* 61: 1363–73.

Thompson, R. (1999). "Early attachment and later development." In J. Cassidy and P. Shaver, (eds). *Handbook of Attachment: Theory, research and clinical applications*. New York: Guilford Press.

Touch the Future Optimum Learning Relationships for Children and Adults. (2004, Spring). 1–16.

Touch Research Institute, Touchpoints, University of Miami, Florida.

Van Boven, S. (1997, Spring/Summer). "Giving infants a helping hand." *Newsweek* Special Issue, 45.

Verney, T., and Kelly, J. (1981). *The Secret Life of the Unborn Child*. New York: Dell.

Warner, J. Mother-child massage helps babies sleep Promotes regular sleep schedule, increses melatonin. www.webmd.com (2004, May 9).

www.birthpsychology.com

Chapter Two

Babeshoff, K.,and Dellinger-Bavolek, J. (1993). *Nurturing Touch*. Park City, Utah: Family Development Resources, Inc.

Barnard, K. (1996). *Beginning Rhythms*. Seattle, WA: NCAST Publications.

Blackburn, S. (1989). "Sleep and awake states of the newborn." In K.E. Barnard (ed.), *Nursing child assessment satellite training resource manual*. Seattle, WA: NCAST Publications.

Brazelton, TB., *Neonatal behavior assessment scale*. Philadelphia: J.B. Lipencott.

Field, T., Schanberg, S., Davalos, M., and Malphurs, J. (1996). "Massage with oil has more positive effects on newborn infants." *Pre and Perinatal Psychology Journal*, 11: 73–78.

Kelly, J., Zuckerman, T., Sandoval, D., and Buehlman, K. (2003). *Promoting First Relationships: A Curriculum for Service Providers to Help Parents and Other Caregivers Meet Young Children's Social and Emotional Needs*. Seattle, WA: NCAST-AVENUW Publications.

McClure, V. (2000). *Infant Massage: A Handbook for Loving Parents*. New York: Bantam.

Schneider, EF. (1995, February). "The role of infant massage in early intervention." Paper presented at the Infant Development Association. San Jose, CA.

Chapter Three

Bartenieff, I. (1970). *Notes from a Course in Correctives*. New York: Dance Notation Bureau.

Bartenieff, I. and Davis, Martha. (1965). *Effort-Shape Analysis of Movement: The Unity of Function and Expression*. New York: Albert Einstein College of Medicine.

DeCasper, A. and Spence, M. Prenatal maternal speech influences newborns' Perception of speech sounds." *Infant Behavior and Development* 9 (1986): 133–150.

Dell, C. *A Primer for Movement Description*. (1970). New York: Dance Notation Bureau, Inc.

Heller, S. (1997). *The Vital Touch*. New York: Henry Holt.

Kestenberg, J. (1965). "The Role of Movement Patterns in Development: 1. Rhythms of Movement." *Psychoanalytic Quarterly*, Vol. XXXIV, No. 1.

Kestenberg, J. (1965). "The Role of Movement Patterns in Development: II The Flow of Tension and Effort. II. The Flow of Tension and Effort." Psychoanalytic Quarterly, Vol. XXXIV, No. 4.

Kestenberg, J. (1967). The Role of Movement Patterns I Development: III. The Control of Shape. *Psychoanalytic Quarterly*, Vol. XXXVI, No. 3.

Laban, R. *Choreutics*. (1966). London: Macdonald and Evans.

Laban, R. and Lawrence, F.C. (1947). *Effort*. London: McDonald and Evans.

Lamb, W. (1965). *Posture and Gesture*. London: Duckworth, 1965.

Macfarlane, A. (1975). "Olfaction in the development of social preferences in the human neonate." *Parent-Infant Interaction*, M. Hofer, (ed). Amsterdam: Elsevier.

Porter, R., Cernoch, J, and McLaughlin, F. "Maternal recognition of neonates through olfactory cues," *Physiology and Behavior* 30 (1985); 151–154.

Weil, A. (1999) *Breathing: The Master Key to Self-Healing*. Louisville, Colorado: Sounds True.

Chapter Four

Brazelton,T., Nugent, J., and Lester, B. (1987). Neonatal behavioral assessment scale. In J.D. Osofsky (Ed.), *Handbook of infant development* (2nd ed.), New Jersey: Wiley.

Chomsky, N. (1957). *Syntactic Structures*. The Hague: Mouton.

De Casper, A., and Spence, M. (1986). "Prenatal maternal speech influences newborn's perception of speech sounds." *Infant Behavior and Development*, 9, 133–150.

Hart, B., and Risley, T. (1995). *Meaningful differences in the everyday experience of young American children*. Baltimore, Maryland: Brookes.

Hepper, P. (1991). "An examination of fetal learning before and after birth." *Irish Journal of Psychology*. 12 (2), 95–107.

Manolson, A. (1992). "It Takes Two To Talk." Toronto: Hanen Early Language Program p. 93.

Olsho, L. "Infant frequency discrimination." *Infant Behavior & Development*, 1984, 7, 27–35.

Salvo, S. (1999). *Massage Therapy*. Pennsylvania: WB Saunders Company.

Santrock, J. (2001). *Child Development*. Boston, Massachusetts: McGraw Hill.

Thorpe, L.A. and Trehub, S. "Duration illusion and auditory grouping in infancy." *Developmental Psychology*, 1989, 25, 122–127.

Trehub, S., Bull, D., and Thorpe, L. "Infants' perception of melodies. The role of melodic contour." *Child Development*, 1984, 55, 821–830.

Tronick,E., Ricks, M., and Cohn, J. (1982), "Maternal and infant affective exchange: patterns of adaptation," in Tiffany Field and Alan Fogel (eds.), *Emotion and Early Interaction, Starting Smart: How Experiences affect brain development.* Hillsdale, New Jersey: Lawrence Erlbaum, 88.

Weinberger, N. (1994/ Spring). The Musical Infant. Musica Research Notes. VI, 17.http://www.musica. uci.edu/mrn/VIIIS94.htl

Chapter Five

Maxwell-Hudson, C. (1988). *The Complete Book of Massage.* New York: Random House.

Chapter Six

American Psychiatric Association. (1994). *Diagnostic and Statistical Manual of Mental Disorders* (4th ed. Rev.). 1994.

Beider, S. (2004) Personal Communication. Integrative Touch Program, Children's Hospital, Los Angeles, California.

Cichetti, D., and Stroufe, A. (1978). "An organizational view of affect. Illustration from the study of Down Syndrome infants." In M. Lewis and L Rosenblum, (eds). *The Development of Affect.* New York: Plenum Press, 309–349.

Commission on Children on Risk. (2004). Hardwired to Connect. The New Scientific Care for Authoritative Communities. New York.

Cullen, L., and Barlow, J. (2002, September). "Kiss, cuddle, squeeze: The experiences and meaning of touch among children with autism attending a touch therapy programme." *Journal of Child Health Care.* 6(3), 171–181.

Drehobl, K., and Fuhr, M. (2000). *Pediatric massage for the child with special needs.* New York: Harcourt Health Sciences.

Educational Resources Information Center. (1998, September). Council on Exceptional Children. Teaching Children with Attention Deficit/Hyperactivity Disorder. ERIC Digest E569.http://www.hoagiesgifted.org/eric/e569.html (2004, September 2)

Escalona, A., Field, T., Singer-Strunck, R., Cullen, C., and Hartshorn, K. (2001). "Autism symptoms decrease following massage therapy." *Journal of Autism and Development.*

Ewart, H. (2002, June). Attention-deficit/hyperactivity disorder: Why massage works. American Massage Therapy Association e-touch. June, 2002.

Feldman, S. (2004). Personal communication. Kaiser Permanente, Woodland Hills, Ca.

Field, T., Hernandez-Reif, M., Quintino, O., Schanberg, S., and Kuhn, C. (1998). "Elder retired volunteers benefit from giving massage therapy to infants." *Journal of Applied Gerontology* 17: 229–239.

Field, T., Lasko, D., Mundy, P., Henteleff, T., Talpins, S., and Dowling, M. (1996). "Autistic children's attentiveness and responsivity improved after touch therapy." *Journal of Autism and Developmental Disorders* 27(3): 333–338.

Field, T., Quintino, O., Hernandez-Reif, M., and Koslovsky, G. (1998). "Adolescents with attention deficit hyperactivity disorder benefit from massage therapy." *Adolescence* 33: 103–108.

Hernandez-Reif, M., Field, T., Largie, S., Diego, M., Manigat, N., Seonanes, J., Bornstein, J., and Waldman, R. (2001). "Cerebral palsy symptoms in children decreased following massage therapy." *Journal of Early Intervention.*

Hernandez-Reif, M., Field, T. and Thimas, E. (2001). "Attention deficit hyperactivity disorder benefit from Tai Chi." *Journal of Body Work and Movement Therapies* 5:120–123.

Hernandez,-Reif, M., Ironson, G., Field, T., Largie, S., Diego, M., Mora,D., Bornstein, J. (2001) "Children with Down Syndrome improved in motor function and muscle tone following massage therapy." *Journal of Early Intervention.*

Hannaford, C. (1995). *Smart Moves Why learning is not all in your head.* Alexander, NC: Great Ocean.

Helliker, B. (2004, October 15) Personal communication. UCLA Hospital, Los Angeles, Ca.

Horowitz, S., Owens, P., & Simms, M. (2000, July). "Specialized Assessments for Children in Foster Care." *Pediatrics,* 106:1 59–67.

Jacobs, R. (2004) Personal Communication. Head of the Division of General Pediatrics Children's Hospital, Los Angeles, CA., and Professor of Pediatrics of Keck School of Medicine, University of Southern California.

Mathias, M., Lowe, J., Ehrhart-Wingard, D. (1998). Touch and massage adaptations for infants born biologically and environmentally at-risk. Course presented by Infant Massage Programs, Albuquerque, New Mexico

McCoy, E. (1985, March) "What's great about grandparents." *Parents,* 65–70.

Meier, G. (1964). "Behavior of infant monkeys, differences attributable to mode of birth," *Science,* 143, 968–970.

Salomonson, J. (2004). Personal communication. Clinical Director, St. John's Hospital, Santa Monica, CA.

Santrock J. (2004) Child Development. (10th ed.), New York:McGraw-Hill.

Schneider, EF. (1999). A Slice of Life. The Learning Channel.

Schneider, E.F. (1997, Fall). Fostering Touch. Tender Loving Care. International Association of Infant Massage. 14(4) 1–3.

Schneider, E.F. (1996, November). Infant Massage and The Power of Touch Enriching Interaction Between Caregivers and Infants. Paper presented at the meeting of the California Governor's Conference Partners in Prevention IV Reaching for Success, Los Angeles, CA.

Schneider, E.F. (1996, January). "The Power of Touch: Massage for Infants." *Infants & Young Children,* 8(3), 40–55.

Sinclair, M. (1992) *Massage for Healthier Children.* Oakland, CA. Wings PW Press.

Simms, M. (1989). "The Foster Care Clinic: A Community Program to Identify Treatment Needs of Children in Foster Care." *Journal of Developmental Behavioral Pediatrics.* 10.

Steinberg, G. (1998). "Bonding and Attachment" How do thoughts effect a newborn? Inside Transitional Pact, An Adoption Alliance www.pactadopt.org (2004, September 10).

Szilagyi. (1998). "The Pediatrician and the Child in Foster Care." *Pediatrics Review,* 19: 39 –50.

Tanghai, J. Baby Constipation. www.netdoctor.co.uk (2004, August 31)

Teaching Children with Attention Deficit/Hyperactivity Disorders ERIC EC Digest 569 www.hoagiesgifted.org/eric/e569.html

Trout, M. (1997). *Multiple Transitions: A Young Child's Point of View on Foster Care and Adoption.* Champaign: Illinois. The Infant-Parent Institute.

Verny, T.and Kelly, J. (1981). *Secret Life of the Unborn Child.* New York: Dell.

Verrier, N. (1998). "Healing the Prime Wound" PACT, An Adoption Alliance www.pactadopt.org (2004, August, 24).

Withers S. (2004, January-February). "Hardwired to Connect." *Twins.* 24–26.

www.chicagorunner.com/twins (2004, September 5)

www.cleftline.org Cleft Palate Foundation, (2004, September 20)

www.commtherapies.com (2004, October 10)

www.drbot.co.uk/club7.20foot.html (2004, September 30)

www.kidshealth.org (2004, September 25)

www.myDNA.com (2004, September 24)

www.nichd.nih.gov/publications/pubs/downsyndrome/down.htm (2004, September 25).

www. spinabifida.us/faz.html (2004, September 11).

www.ucp.org (2004, September 29)

Conclusion

Calvert, R. *The History of Massage.* (2002). Rochester, Vermont: Healing Arts Press.

Kelly, J., Zuckerman, T., Sandoval, D., and Buehlman, K. (2003). *Promoting First Relationships: A Curriculum for Service Providers to Help Parents and Other Caregivers Meet Young Children's Social and Emotional Needs.* Seattle, WA: NCAST-AVENUW Publications.

Shore, R. (1997). *Rethinking the Brain.* New York: Families and Work Institute.

ABOUT THE AUTHOR

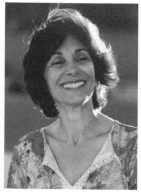

Elaine Fogel Schneider holds a PhD in psychology as well as master of arts degrees in the fields of speech-language pathology and dance/movement therapy. She is certified as an instructor of infant massage and is a certified group psychotherapist. She is also a faculty member in the California State University system's psychology department, and a governor appointee to the State of California's Interagency Coordinating Council for infants, toddlers, and their families.

Dr. Schneider is the founder of Baby Steps, a comprehensive family-focused early intervention program, and Community Therapies, which provides multidisciplinary programs for hundreds of infants, toddlers, and children with developmental disabilities and at-risk conditions. Community Therapies has been named a Center of Excellence with the Los Angeles County Department of Mental Health.

As one of the leading experts in the country on infant massage, Dr. Schneider has presented for organizations such as Zero to Three, International Association of Infant Massage, UNESCO, Head Start, Early Head Start, Infant Development Association of California, and the Center for the Improvement of Child Caring, as well as for major school districts and preschools throughout the country and world.

Dr. Schneider's articles have been published in national professional journals, *Massage Magazine,* and other periodicals, and have been referenced in textbooks and infant massage books. Dr. Schneider's article "The Power of Touch: Massage for Infants" first appeared in the peer-reviewed journal *Infants and Young Children* (1996) and laid the foundation for using infant massage in many early-intervention birth-to-three programs throughout the country.

Dr. Schneider was featured on the Learning Channel's national cable television program *Slice of Life.* She is also a California Department of Education Consultant for the SEEDS (Supporting Early Education Delivery Systems) Project.

The co-author of *Pictures Please,* Dr. Elaine Fogel Schneider is a wife and mother and lives in the Los Angeles area. You can visit her website at www.askdrelaine.com.

℘HOTO ℭREDITS

Edo Tsoar: pages 21, 24, 31, 52, 62, 93 (lower), 94 (Pat-A-Foot and Jumping Jacks), 97 (top), 127, 131, 136, 138, 140 (top), 144, and 147.

Karen B. Christy: pages 9, 10, 11, 14, 15, 16, 22, 28, 32, 33, 34, 44, 51, 53, 54, 59, 60, 61, 63, 64, 66, 67, 68, 69, 70, 71, 72, 73, 74, 75, 76, 77, 79, 80, 82, 83, 84, 86, 87, 88, 89, 90, 93 (upper), 94 (Bicycle Built for Two), 95, 96, 97 (bottom), 102, 103, 105, 137, 140 (bottom), 148, 163, 164, 167, 169, 172, 176, 178, 181, 184, 185, 186, and 192.

$\mathcal{I}$NDEX

OTHER SQUAREONE TITLES OF INTEREST

THE GENTLE REVOLUTION SERIES

The Institutes for the Achievement of Human Potential has been successfully serving children and teaching parents for five decades. Its goal has been to significantly improve the intellectual, physical, and social development of all children. The groundbreaking methods and techniques of the Institutes have set the standards in early childhood education. As a result, the books written by Glenn Doman, founder of this organization, have become the all-time best-selling parenting series in the United States—and the world. With over 12 million copies of these books in print, and the demand continuing to grow, Square One is proud to be the new publisher of this phenomenal series of at-home teaching titles.

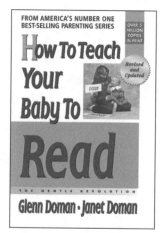

$13.95 US / $20.95 CAN • paper
ISBN 0-7570-0185-8

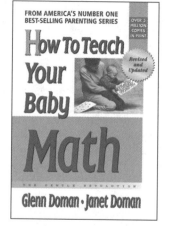

$13.95 US / $20.95 CAN • paper
ISBN 0-7570-0184-X

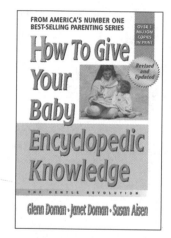

$13.95 US / $20.95 CAN • paper
ISBN 0-7570-0182-3

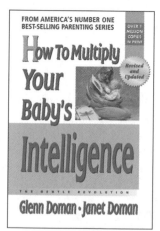

$15.95 US / $23.95 CAN • paper
ISBN 0-7570-0183-1

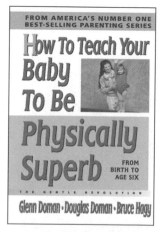

$29.95 US / $44.95 CAN • cloth
ISBN 0-7570-0192-0

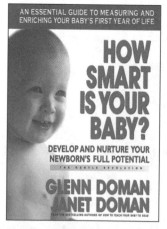

$16.95 US / $22.95 CAN • paper
ISBN 0-7570-0194-7

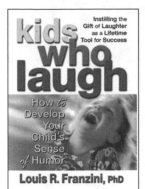

KIDS WHO LAUGH
How to Develop Your Child's Sense of Humor
Louis R. Franzini, PhD

While some children are born with a sense of humor, for most kids, humor is a learned behavior. Unfortunately, most parents never really focus on this important characteristic, and have no idea how to instill it in their children. *Kids Who Laugh* is the first book to examine the many benefits humor has to offer, including self-confidence, coping skills, self-control, and more. Most important, it offers the actual tools that parents can use to develop a child's healthy and abiding sense of humor.

$14.95 US / $22.50 CAN • 192 pages • 6 x 9-inch quality paperback • ISBN 0-7570-0008-8

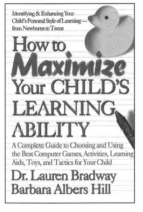

HOW TO MAXIMIZE YOUR CHILD'S LEARNING ABILITY
A Complete Guide to Choosing and Using the Best Computer Games, Activities, Learning Aids, Toys, and Tactics for Your Child
Dr. Lauren Bradway and Barbara Albers Hill

Over twenty years ago, Dr. Lauren Bradway discovered that all children have specific learning styles. Some learn best through visual stimulation; others, through sound and language; and still others, through touch. In *How to Maximize Your Child's Learning Ability*, Dr. Bradway first shows you how to determine your child's inherent style. She then aids you in carefully selecting the toys, activities, and educational strategies that will help reinforce the talents and traits your child was born with, and encourage those skills that come less easily.

$14.95 US / $23.95 CAN • 288 pages • 6 x 9-inch quality paperback • ISBN 0-7570-0096-7

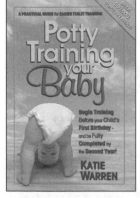

POTTY TRAINING YOUR BABY
A Practical Guide for Easier Toilet Training
Katie Warren

Potty Training Your Baby includes information on everything from where to buy a potty to dealing with those inevitable little "accidents." The material is presented in a down-to-earth fashion, and is enhanced by the author's personal parenting experiences. Perhaps most important, the author shows you how to turn this often dreaded and frustrating task into a time of growth and learning for both you and your child.

$9.95 US / $14.95 CAN • 104 pages • 6 x 9-inch quality paperback • ISBN 0-7570-0180-7